Musculoskeletal Examination
of the
Elbow, Wrist, and Hand

Making the Complex Simple

Randall W. Culp, MD
The Philadelphia and South Jersey Hand Centers
Philadelphia, Pennsylvania

Sidney M. Jacoby, MD
The Philadelphia and South Jersey Hand Centers
Philadelphia, Pennsylvania

MUSCULOSKELETAL EXAMINATION
MAKING THE COMPLEX SIMPLE
SERIES

Series Editor, Steven B. Cohen, MD

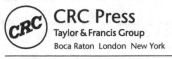

CRC Press
Taylor & Francis Group
Boca Raton London New York

CRC Press is an imprint of the
Taylor & Francis Group, an **Informa** business

First published 2012 by SLACK Incorporated

Published 2024 by CRC Press
2385 NW Executive Center Drive, Suite 320, Boca Raton FL 33431

and by CRC Press
4 Park Square, Milton Park, Abingdon, Oxon, OX14 4RN

CRC Press is an imprint of Taylor & Francis Group, LLC

© 2012 Taylor & Francis Group, LLC

Library of Congress Cataloging-in-Publication Data

Musculoskeletal examination of the elbow, wrist, and hand : making the complex simple / edited by Randall W. Culp, Sidney M. Jacoby.
   p. ; cm. -- (Musculoskeletal examination series)
 Includes bibliographical references and index.
  ISBN 978-1-55642-918-7 (alk. paper)
 I. Culp, Randall W. II. Jacoby, Sidney M. III. Series: Musculoskeletal examination : making the complex simple series.
  [DNLM: 1. Elbow Joint--injuries. 2. Hand Injuries--diagnosis. 3. Musculoskeletal Diseases--diagnosis. 4. Physical Examination--methods. 5. Wrist Injuries--diagnosis. WE 820]
  LC classification not assigned
  617.4'72044--dc23
                          2011045048
ISBN: 9781556429187 (pbk)
ISBN: 9781003525103 (ebk)

DOI: 10.1201/9781003525103

DEDICATION

Thank you to my wife, Beth, for your love, encouragement, and patience.
Randall W. Culp, MD

To my loving wife and beautiful children.
You are the joys of my life.
SMJ

CONTENTS

Dedication iii
Acknowledgments vi
About the Editors vii
Contributing Authors ix
Introduction xii

SECTION I PHYSICAL EXAMINATION 1

Chapter 1   Physical Examination of the Elbow: The Basics
             and Specific Tests 2
             Taruna Madhav Crawford, MD and
             Uzoma Ukomadu, MD

Chapter 2   Physical Examination of the Wrist: The Basics
             and Specific Tests 14
             Brandon J. Valentine, MD and Randall W. Culp, MD

Chapter 3   Physical Examination of the Hand: The Basics
             and Specific Tests 36
             John J. Fernandez, MD, FAAOS

SECTION II GENERAL IMAGING 72

Chapter 4   General Imaging of the Elbow 73
             Hiu Yan Miranda Lai, MBChB, FRCR, MMed;
             Amy F. Austin, MD; Kristen E. McClure, MD; and
             William B. Morrison, MD

Chapter 5   General Imaging of the Wrist 95
             Frank E. Mullens, MD, MPH and
             William B. Morrison, MD

Chapter 6   General Imaging of the Hand 121
             John Shum Sing Fai, MBBS, FRCR and
             William B. Morrison, MD

SECTION III COMMON CONDITIONS OF THE ELBOW, WRIST, AND HAND 138

Chapter 7   Elbow Instability 139
             Min Jung Park, MD, MMSc and Jeffrey Yao, MD

Chapter 8   Ligament Injuries of the Wrist and Hand 159
             Danielle Scher, MD and Jennifer Moriatis Wolf, MD

Chapter 9   Neuropathy 183
             Jason M. Erpelding, MD and Anthony J. Lauder, MD

Chapter 10   Common Tendinopathies of the Wrist
             and Elbow.. 212
             David Essig, MD and Seth D. Dodds, MD

Chapter 11   Ulnar Wrist: Triangular Fibrocartilage Complex
             and Distal Radio-Ulnar Joint............................228
             Min Jung Park, MD, MMSc and Jeffrey Yao, MD

Chapter 12   Arthritis of the Elbow, Wrist, and Hand 252
             Brian D. Adams, MD

Chapter 13   Examination of Elbow, Wrist, and Hand
             Fractures 274
             David Ring, MD, PhD

Chapter 14   Wounds and Soft-Tissue Injuries 291
             Jeffrey B. Friedrich, MD, FACS

Chapter 15   Vascular Evaluation of the Upper Extremity.. 310
             Diane Payne, MD and Marc J. Richard, MD

Financial Disclosures..*328*
Index *330*

ACKNOWLEDGMENTS

Thanks to Carli Lontz, my secretary.
Randall W. Culp, MD

About the Editors

Randall W. Culp, MD, is a member of the prestigious Philadelphia Hand Center. Born in Wheeling, West Virginia, Dr. Culp attended the College of William & Mary and received his medical degree from Penn State University. While at the University of Pennsylvania, Dr. Culp was selected for a Surgical Internship, Residencies in Orthopedic Surgical Research and Orthopedic Surgery, and a Post-Residency Hand Surgery Fellowship.

Dr. Culp was named one of the area's "Top Doctors" in the field of hand surgery by *Philadelphia* magazine, and has received numerous awards for performance and research. He is the recipient of the George B. Archer Award (chemistry student at William & Mary), the Upjohn Award (excellence in creative scholarship at Penn State), the Deforest Willard Award (outstanding performance, University of Pennsylvania), the Meyerding Award (excellence in fracture care), the Navy Achievement Medal (service in the Persian Gulf War), and the Humanitarian Service Medal (service during the San Francisco earthquake).

He is currently Professor of Orthopaedic, Hand, and Microsurgery at Thomas Jefferson University, and serves on the board of the Hand Rehabilitation Foundation. He has served on the council of the American Society for Surgery of the Hand and is now on the board of the American College of Surgeons. In addition, he is the consulting hand and wrist surgeon to the Philadelphia Phillies baseball organization, as well as the Philadelphia Flyers hockey organization.

Recognizing the importance of giving back, Dr. Culp participates yearly in medical missions, bringing his services to international communities. He is committed to delivering state-of-the-art care for the hand, wrist, elbow, and arm to his patients. Dr. Culp is integrally involved in breakthrough research and regularly shares his expertise through numerous publications and presentations.

Sidney M. Jacoby, MD, is a member of the renowned Philadelphia Hand Center at Thomas Jefferson University Hospital. Originally from Atlantic City, New Jersey, Dr. Jacoby graduated with honors from The University of Pennsylvania. He obtained his medical degree from Jefferson Medical College in Philadelphia. While at Jefferson, he completed his orthopaedic surgery training and pursued additional sub-specialty training in hand, wrist, and elbow surgery at The Philadelphia Hand Center. Subsequently, Dr. Jacoby joined The Philadelphia Hand Center and is currently Assistant Professor of Orthopaedic Surgery at Thomas Jefferson University Hospital. He is also Chief of Hand Surgery at Phoenixville Hospital and the Clinical Research Coordinator of the Philadelphia Hand Center.

Dr. Jacoby has been recognized throughout his academic career for both scholastic excellence and a genuine devotion to patient care. As an undergraduate student at University of Pennsylvania, Dr. Jacoby was awarded multiple government sponsored research fellowships at The National Institutes of Health (NIH) in Bethesda, Maryland. At Jefferson Medical College, he was awarded the prestigious James D. and Jennie M. Beach Memorial Scholarship, which provided a full academic scholarship for outstanding academic performance and an extraordinary commitment to the Jefferson community. As an orthopaedic resident, Dr. Jacoby was awarded The Mark D. Chilton Award, which recognized an outstanding level of compassion and commitment to patients entrusted to his care, as well as The Philip Syng Physick Annual Award, honoring orthopaedic residents with the most outstanding senior research project.

As an avid researcher, Dr. Jacoby has already authored numerous scientific and clinical publications. Dr. Jacoby's commitment to academic medicine and patient care are guiding principles that he inherited from his outstanding mentors. Dr. Jacoby loves spending time with his young family, including his two children and neurosurgeon wife. He also likes to travel and enjoy Philadelphia's rich culture and history.

CONTRIBUTING AUTHORS

Brian D. Adams, MD (Chapter 12)
Department of Orthopedic Surgery
University of Iowa
Iowa City, Iowa

Amy F. Austin, MD (Chapter 4)
Attending Radiologist
Atlantic Medical Imaging
Galloway, New Jersey

Taruna Madhav Crawford, MD (Chapter 1)
MidAmerica Orthopaedics Hand to Shoulder Clinic
Oakbrook Terrace, Illinois

Seth D. Dodds, MD (Chapter 10)
Assistant Professor, Hand and Upper Extremity Surgery
Department of Orthopaedics and Rehabilitation
Yale University School of Medicine
New Haven, Connecticut

Jason M. Erpelding, MD (Chapter 9)
Hand Surgery Fellow
Medical College of Wisconsin
Milwaukee, Wisconsin

David Essig, MD (Chapter 10)
Chief Resident, Orthopaedic Surgery
Yale University
New Haven, Connecticut

John Shum Sing Fai, MBBS, FRCR (Chapter 6)
Pamela Youde Nethersole Eastern Hospital
Hong Kong, China

John J. Fernandez, MD, FAAOS (Chapter 3)
Associate Professor of Orthopaedic Surgery
Rush University Medical Center
Chicago, Illinois

Jeffrey B. Friedrich, MD, FACS (Chapter 14)
University of Washington
Seattle, Washington

Hiu Yan Miranda Lai, MBChB, FRCR, MMed (Chapter 4)
United Christian Hospital
Kwun Tong, Hong Kong, China

Anthony J. Lauder, MD (Chapter 9)
Hand & Wrist Surgery
Longview Orthopedic Associates
Longview, Washington

Kristen E. McClure, MD (Chapter 4)
Thomas Jefferson University Hospital
Philadelphia, Pennsylvania

William B. Morrison, MD (Chapters 4, 5, 6)
Thomas Jefferson University Hospital
Philadelphia, Pennsylvania

Frank E. Mullens, MD, MPH (Chapter 5)
Walter Reed National Military Medical Center
Bethesda, Maryland

Min Jung Park, MD, MMSc (Chapters 7, 11)
Instructor B
Perelman School of Medicine, University of Pennsylvania
Department of Orthopedic Surgery, Hospitals of the
University of Pennsylvania
Philadelphia, Pennsylvania

Diane Payne, MD (Chapter 15)
Duke University Medical Center
Durham, North Carolina

Marc J. Richard, MD (Chapter 15)
Duke University Medical Center
Durham, North Carolina

David Ring, MD, PhD (Chapter 13)
Massachusetts General Hospital
Boston, Massachusetts

Danielle Scher, MD (Chapter 8)
William Beaumont Army Medical Center
El Paso, Texas

Uzoma Ukomadu, MD (Chapter 1)
Thomas Jefferson University Hospital
Philadelphia, Pennsylvania

Brandon J. Valentine, MD (Chapter 2)
Barron & Homesley Orthopedic Specialists
Charlotte, North Carolina

Jennifer Moriatis Wolf, MD (Chapter 8)
University of Connecticut Health Center
Farmington, Connecticut

Jeffrey Yao, MD (Chapters 7, 11)
Stanford University
Palo Alto, California

INTRODUCTION

The physical examination of the elbow, wrist, and hand represents the most elemental form of patient evaluation, but it can often challenge even the most experienced health care provider. In what is justly considered an advanced era of health care delivery, the art of the physical examination has regrettably been usurped by a reliance on advanced imaging and other diagnostic indicators. Many believe that the art of the musculoskeletal examination has eroded, and as a result, the sacred physician-patient encounter has been compromised.

With this thought in mind, *Musculoskeletal Examination of the Elbow, Wrist, and Hand: Making the Complex Simple* is an attempt to revisit the basics of the physical examination and reacquaint the reader with the crucial elements of a thorough upper extremity evaluation. Inside this pocket-sized book, you will find an inclusive guide to a complete review of the most common pathologic conditions, the techniques for accurate diagnosis, as well as treatment pearls. This book includes sections not only on physical examination, but also on diagnostic imaging and the care of upper extremity fractures and soft tissue pathology.

Musculoskeletal Examination of the Elbow, Wrist, and Hand: Making the Complex Simple takes complex subject matter and distills it to an easily understood, reproducible, and enjoyable experience that will be welcomed by orthopedic residents, attendings, physical therapists, athletic trainers, medical students, or anyone interested in sharpening their diagnostic and therapeutic skill set.

We hope you enjoy learning and implementing your new skills as much as we have enjoyed arranging the material in this "handy" little book.

Randall W. Culp, MD and Sidney M. Jacoby, MD

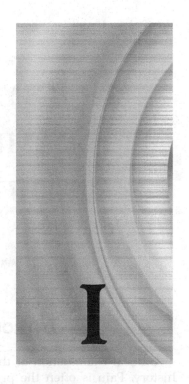

I

Physical Examination

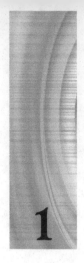

1

PHYSICAL EXAMINATION OF THE ELBOW
THE BASICS AND SPECIFIC TESTS

Taruna Madhav Crawford, MD and Uzoma Ukomadu, MD

INTRODUCTION

Clinical examination of the elbow begins with a detailed history. Pain is often the presenting symptom and may be due to a number of causes. The examiner must note the onset, chronicity, and quality of the symptoms. Current symptoms may be related to an acute injury or remote trauma, such as an injury during childhood. Congenital syndromes, especially those with mild manifestations, may not become symptomatic

Culp RW, Jacoby SM. *Musculoskeletal Examination of the Elbow, Wrist, and Hand: Making the Complex Simple* (pp. 2-13). © 2012 Taylor & Francis Group.

until later in life. Additionally—as there is often overlapping symptomatology with conditions of the cervical spine, shoulder, elbow, wrist, and hand—it is important to inquire about adjacent joint discomfort. A thorough and detailed history will make the physical examination more specific to the etiology of the patient's symptoms. It will also help establish a rapport with the patient, so that the patient may more accurately communicate during the physical examination.

PHYSICAL EXAMINATION

After obtaining a thorough history, start with inspection of both elbows. Ask the patient to remove any clothing or jewelry that may obscure anatomic landmarks. This is also an appropriate time to perform an examination of the neck, bilateral shoulders, bilateral wrists, and bilateral hands, as elbow symptoms may be a manifestation of pathology elsewhere in the neck or upper extremity.

Visual Inspection

On initial examination of the elbow, notice the skin and the surrounding soft tissues. Note any scars from prior trauma or surgery. Assess for any signs of recent trauma such as swelling, ecchymosis, or abrasions. Note any localized joint swelling, which may appear in the soft spots along the elbow—the posterior soft spot formed by the posterior aspect of the ulnohumeral joint or a lateral soft spot formed in the triangle of the olecranon, radial head, and lateral epicondyle (Figure 1-1). Masses, nodules, or tophi, especially on the extensor surface, may indicate inflammatory conditions or gout. Psoriatic lesions also may be present on the extensor surface and may appear as gray-white scales. Note any erythema or edema of the extremity, which would indicate infection. In patients with prior corticosteroid injection, there may be subcutaneous atrophy or skin pigmentation changes at the injection site. Asymmetrical venous dilation of the basilic or cephalic veins may be indicative of a venous thoracic outlet syndrome. Diffuse swelling of the arm may indicate venous disorder or lymphedema. The ulnar nerve in thinner individuals may be

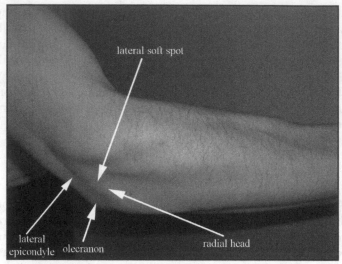

Figure 1-1. Soft spots along elbow.

visible and may demonstrate subluxation over the medial epicondyle with elbow extension and flexion.

Compare the involved side with the uninvolved side in regard to muscle atrophy or hypertrophy. A measurement of the circumference of the arm 7 cm distal to the prominent medial epicondyle may help in identifying subtle differences. Atrophy of the mobile wad of three (the brachioradialis, extensor carpi radialis brevis, and extensor carpi radialis longus) may indicate a high radial nerve injury (Figure 1-2). The biceps tendon may be less prominent in the antecubital fossa, and the patient may have a more prominent biceps muscle in a proximal or distal biceps tendon rupture.

Much of the bony anatomy is readily visible about the elbow. Bony deformity or asymmetry in the carrying angle of the elbow should be noted. A normal carrying angle of the elbow is on average 10 degrees for men and 13 degrees for women (Figure 1-3). The olecranon tip is visible subcutaneously. An increased prominence may indicate posterior elbow subluxation, an enthesopathy, or triceps rupture. Decreased prominence may indicate anterior elbow subluxation. A prominent medial epicondyle may contribute to snapping triceps syndrome or ulnar neuropathy.

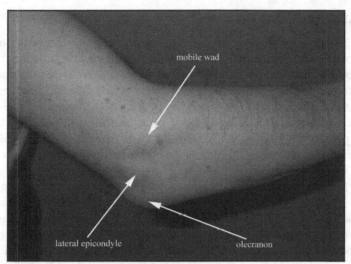

mobile wad

lateral epicondyle   olecranon

Figure 1-2. Atrophy of the mobile wad of three may indicate a high radial nerve injury.

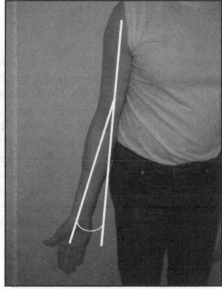

Figure 1-3. The normal carrying angle of the elbow is on average 10 degrees for men and 13 degrees for women.

Range of Motion

At the next stage of the examination, evaluate the range of motion of both elbows. Measure the degrees of extension to flexion, noting any hyperextension or contractures. Normal range of motion at the elbow is approximately 0 to 150 degrees, with a functional range of motion of 30 to 130 degrees for most activities of daily living. Elbow pronation and supination is approximately 80 to 90 degrees in each direction, with most functional activities being able to be performed with an arc of 50 degrees of pronation and 50 degrees of supination.

Note any discrepancy between active and passive range of motion, which may indicate tendon injury or weakness due to neurologic etiology. Also determine whether the end point is soft or hard. Although a hard end point may indicate a bony block, significant contracture will also often result in a hard end point from the contracted joint capsule. Limitations in pronation and supination may be secondary to the distal radioulnar joint or proximal radioulnar joint. A congenital or post-traumatic change in the radial bow or ulnar shaft alignment or length may also limit rotation.

Palpation

Until this point in the examination, the patient has become accustomed to describing symptoms and demonstrating the elbow to the examiner. An accurate examination of the elbow after this point depends on experience, expediency, and an appropriate order in approaching the examination. Frequently, patients will point out the most symptomatic aspect of the elbow. It is prudent to consider the differential diagnosis and examine this aspect last in terms of palpation or provocative maneuvers.

Begin with palpation of the bony prominences. Palpate the medial epicondyle, olecranon, lateral condyle, and radial head. The olecranon fossa and posteromedial ulnohumeral joint may be palpated by maximally flexing the elbow. Medial epicondyle or lateral condyle pain may be present with epicondylitis. An occult trauma to the radial head may be differentiated by tenderness to palpation. Tenderness along the posterior olecranon and triceps insertion may be present in posterior elbow impingement or valgus extension overload syndrome. In thin

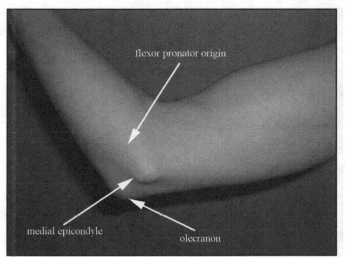

Figure 1-4. Tenderness at the origin of the flexor pronator mass may be elicited with medial epicondylitis.

patients, the radial tuberosity may also be palpated; the posterior interosseous nerve is just distal to the tuberosity.

Palpate the origins or insertions of the muscles about the elbow. As previously stated, pain about the distal triceps may be due to valgus extension overload. Pain over the triceps with deformity and loss of elbow extension may represent a triceps avulsion or proximal olecranon fracture. Tenderness over the origin of the extensor carpi radialis brevis may demonstrate lateral epicondylitis. On the medial aspect of the elbow, a snapping band of the triceps may be palpable and may cause medial-sided elbow pain. Tenderness at the origin of the flexor pronator mass may be elicited with medial epicondylitis (Figure 1-4). The biceps tendon insertion at the anterior elbow may be palpated and the index finger hooked about the tendon (Figure 1-5). In a distal biceps tendon rupture, this tendon may not be hooked; in a biceps tendon rupture, the lacertus fibrosis may be mistaken for the biceps tendon.

Nerve pathology may also be tactile. Palpation over the ulnar nerve while the elbow is flexed and extended may demonstrate ulnar nerve subluxation. A Tinel's sign may be present by tapping on the ulnar nerve, causing paresthesias down the

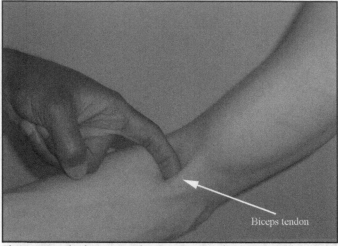
Biceps tendon

Figure 1-5. The biceps tendon insertion at the anterior elbow may be palpated and the index finger hooked about the tendon.

medial arm into the small and ring fingers. A Tinel's sign may also be performed to evaluate for radial tunnel syndrome by tapping on the radial nerve as it passes under the supinator muscle, causing paresthesias along the volar forearm without any muscle weakness. Pronator syndrome, causing paresthesias or numbness of the thumb, index, middle, and lateral aspect of the ring finger as well as palmar symptoms, may be determined by tenderness or a positive Tinel's sign along the anterior forearm at the pronator arcade.

Strength Testing

Strength testing of the elbow may be performed to evaluate flexion, extension, pronation, and supination. Pronation and supination may be tested by having the patient place the elbow at the side with the elbow flexed to 90 degrees and forearm in neutral position. The examiner should use one hand to stabilize the arm and the second hand to grasp the patient's hand, asking the patient to rotate against resistance. Strength is graded on a scale of 0 to 5 and is compared with the contralateral elbow.

Grip and pinch strength may also be useful to quantify, especially after neuropathy or tendon pathology. Grip strength testing may be performed with a hand dynamometer, with the elbows adducted to the side and unsupported. The elbow should be flexed to 90 degrees, the forearm placed in neutral position, and the wrist dorsiflexed between 0 and 30 degrees and ulnarly deviated between 0 and 15 degrees. Maximal grip strength is usually at the second or third setting, and single-setting testing is frequently performed at the second setting. Key and tip pinch testing may also be evaluated, especially for patients with neuropathy.

Provocative Maneuver/Special Tests

Tendonitis may be elicited with resisted motion recreating the patient's pain. Medial epicondylitis may be differentiated from pronator syndrome by resisted forearm pronation and wrist flexion, creating pain directly over the medial epicondyle as opposed to along the forearm in pronator syndrome. Resisted forearm supination and wrist extension may recreate symptoms of lateral epicondylitis. Resisted elbow extension may recreate symptoms of triceps tendonitis or valgus extension overload.

Ulnar neuropathy at the elbow may be provoked by elbow hyperflexion and compression along the medial elbow. Firm pressure held over the pronator arcade or hyperflexion and pronation of the forearm may be used to assess for pronator syndrome. Radial tunnel syndrome, often confused with lateral epicondylitis, may be differentiated by pressure over the supinator muscle causing volar arm pain. As it is not accompanied by muscle weakness, it may be differentiated by posterior interosseous nerve syndrome, which causes wrist and digital weakness without pain.

Stability testing is a very important aspect of the examination. Symptoms of medial instability, as may be seen in throwing athletes, may be evaluated with the valgus extension overload test. Begin with the elbow flexed, and maintain a valgus stress on the elbow while taking it into extension (Figure 1-6). Pain or medial opening along the posteromedial aspect of the olecranon may be due to ulnar collateral ligament incompetence. The patient may also have a positive "milking maneuver," where the elbow is flexed to 90 degrees, the

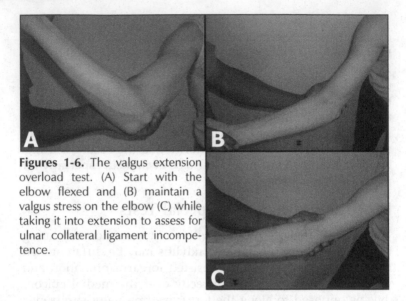

Figures 1-6. The valgus extension overload test. (A) Start with the elbow flexed and (B) maintain a valgus stress on the elbow (C) while taking it into extension to assess for ulnar collateral ligament incompetence.

forearm is fully supinated, and the hand is made into a fist with the thumb abducted. The patient's contralateral arm is then crossed anteriorly to the tested arm, and the thumb is pulled laterally, placing a valgus stress on the elbow (Figure 1-7). Pain with this test demonstrates incompetence of the anterior band of the ulnar collateral ligament complex. The posterior aspect of the ulnar collateral ligament complex may be best stressed by placing the elbow in 30 degrees of flexion to unlock the olecranon and placing valgus stress. In thinner patients with less subcutaneous fat, the origin of the medial collateral ligament complex may also be palpated while performing provocative maneuvers. The anterior oblique portion of the medial collateral ligament is the primary valgus stabilizer of the elbow. Often, medial instability may also stress the radiocapitellar joint, causing chondromalacia. This may be tested during the valgus extension overload test, or also with pronation and supination of the forearm with the elbow in flexion to assess for radiocapitellar pain or crepitus.

The elbow may be assessed for posterolateral instability, which is present when there is deficiency of the lateral ulnar collateral ligament. The pivot shift test is performed with the

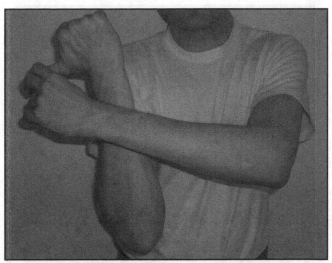

Figure 1-7. The milking maneuver.

forearm fully supinated and the elbow extended. The elbow is then slowly flexed while placing axial compression and maintaining a supination and valgus force at the elbow. In posterolateral instability, this may elicit pain along the posterolateral elbow or cause subluxation of the ulnohumeral joint while the elbow is extended and reduction of the joint when it reaches approximately 40 degrees (Figure 1-8). Because this is painful, it may create apprehension in awake patients. In a patient under anesthesia, a clunk is felt at reduction. The tabletop relocation test is a provocative maneuver that attempts to recreate the pain or weakness that patients with posterolateral instability may experience with pushing up through the elbow, such as with pushing up from a chair. The forearm is placed in supination on a tabletop with the hand hanging off the edge of the table. The forearm is loaded, and the elbow is allowed to flex. In posterolateral instability, symptoms are recreated at approximately 40 degrees as the radial head subluxates posteriorly. This maneuver is repeated with the examiner's thumb firmly pressing on the radial head; the patient may not be as symptomatic this second time. However, by removing the pressure along the radial head in this position, the symptoms are recreated as they were in the first attempt.

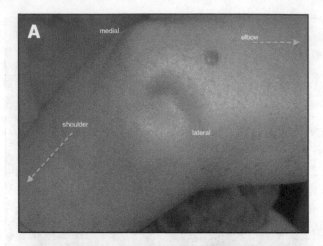

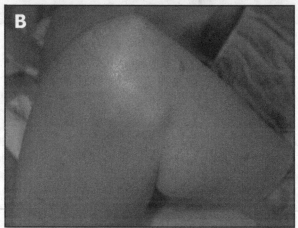

Figure 1-8. Posterolateral rotatory instability. (A) A dimple is seen on the lateral aspect of the elbow as the ulno-humeral joint is subluxed under pivot shift testing in extension. (B) The dimple disappears as the joint reduces in flexion. (Reprinted with permission of Dr. Phani Dantuluri.)

CONCLUSION

Although the elbow examination may seem fairly complex, a combination of a thorough history and physical examination will frequently identify the source of pathology. The key is to develop a differential diagnosis from the patient's history and then perform an examination in a systematic order, making certain to visually inspect palpation, strength testing, and provocative maneuvers that may increase the patient's symptoms near the end of the examination. Supportive imaging studies will also be useful but will be more useful if the appropriate differential diagnosis is formulated prior to ordering the study. A thorough and focused clinical examination is possible through patience, application for the range of pathologies possible, practice, and—ultimately—experience.

SUGGESTED READING

Arvind C, Hargreaves D. Table top relocation test—New clinical test for posterolateral rotatory instability of the elbow. *J Should Elbow Surg.* 2006;15(4):500-501.

Colman WW, Strauch RJ. Physical examination of the elbow. *Orthop Clin North Am.* 1999;30(1):15-20.

O'Driscoll SW, Bell DF, Morrey BF. Posterolateral rotatory instability of the elbow. *J Bone Joint Surg.* 1991;73A:440-446.

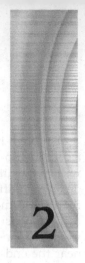

2

PHYSICAL EXAMINATION OF THE WRIST
THE BASICS AND SPECIFIC TESTS

Brandon J. Valentine, MD and Randall W. Culp, MD

INTRODUCTION

A thorough and accurate history and physical examination are essential in the diagnosis and management of the painful wrist. A skilled clinician can derive more useful information from a well-performed examination than from any available imaging study. While radiographs and more advanced imaging can serve as a valuable adjunct in confirming a diagnosis

Culp RW, Jacoby SM. *Musculoskeletal Examination of the Elbow, Wrist, and Hand: Making the Complex Simple* (pp. 14-35). © 2012 Taylor & Francis Group.

and defining the extent of pathology, a diligent history and clinical examination form the cornerstone of evaluation and management.

HISTORY

Eliciting a thorough and focused history can be one of the most challenging tasks for a clinician. Properly executed, it can yield a wealth of valuable information for the diagnosis and management of wrist conditions. A complete history includes the date of onset or duration of symptoms, details of any precipitating incident or activities, position of the wrist during injury, and subsequent degree and direction of stress. Patient description of the location, intensity, and duration of symptoms, along with activities and positions that aggravate or relieve symptoms, should be recorded. Any prior treatments or studies and improvement or worsening of symptoms over time are noted. Finally, the overall impact of the condition on the patient's daily living, leisure and athletic pursuits, and ability to work are assessed. Information obtained from the patient's history helps to focus the physical examination and serves as the background in which the examination findings are interpreted.

INSPECTION/PALPATION

Simple observation of the patient upon entering the examination room can provide useful information. We do not routinely offer to shake hands, as most patients have hand and wrist complaints. The patient who offers to shake and does so with a firm grip is telling us that he or she continues to use his or her dominant hand and wrist well for simple daily activities. Observe the posture of the hand; note any areas of swelling, nodules, or masses; identify any erythema, abrasions, and previous surgical incisions; and record their location and size. Measure active range of motion (AROM) and passive range of motion (PROM) bilaterally, and ask the patient to point to the area of maximal pain. Palpate bony prominences and soft tissue anatomy to further define areas of tenderness and localize any crepitus, clicks, or clunks the patient reports being able to produce.

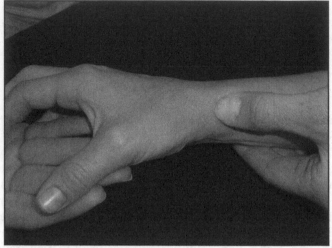

Figure 2-1. Palpation of the radial styloid.

TOPOGRAPHIC EXAMINATION

After initial inspection and palpation is complete, a more focused systematic examination is performed, evaluating the 5 topographic zones described by Lichtman. Specific maneuvers and tests are used in each zone to define regional pathology:

- Radial dorsal zone
- Central dorsal zone
- Ulnar dorsal zone
- Radial volar zone
- Ulnar volar zone

Radial Dorsal Zone

The radial dorsal zone is a common site of wrist pain from trauma, tendonitis, and arthritic conditions. Evaluation in the radial dorsal zone begins with the radial styloid, palpating proximal to the snuffbox with the wrist in ulnar deviation (Figure 2-1). Tenderness here may indicate contusion, fracture, or radioscaphoid arthritis. The latter is common with

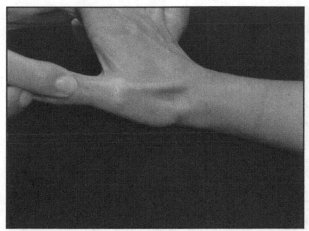

Figure 2-2. Radial snuffbox between the first and third dorsal extensor compartments.

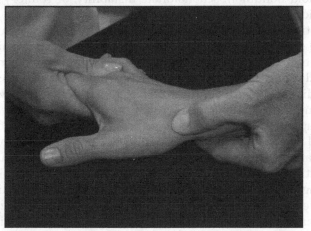

Figure 2-3. Palpation of the scaphoid within the snuffbox.

longstanding scapholunate (SL) dissociation. Tenderness may be accentuated with radial deviation.

Distal to the radial styloid, the snuffbox (Figure 2-2) is identified between the extensor pollicis longus (EPL) and the first extensor compartment tendons, the abductor pollicis longus (APL), and extensor pollicis brevis (EPB). With the wrist in ulnar deviation, palpation of the snuffbox isolates the scaphoid (Figure 2-3). Tenderness here may indicate scaphoid fracture,

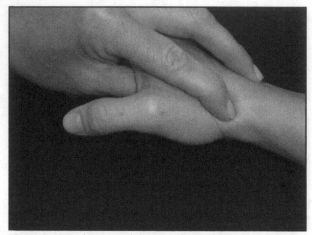

Figure 2-4. Palpation of the thumb CMC joint.

scaphoid nonunion, scapholunate instability, or rotatory sub-luxation of the scaphoid.

Activities requiring repetitive wrist hyperextension can cause radial dorsal wrist pain. Gymnast's wrist is a painful condition caused by proximal scaphoid impingement on the dorsal rim of the distal radius with repetitive contact. Consider this diagnosis with reproduction of radial dorsal pain when loading the hyperextended wrist.

Scaphotrapezial (ST) joint arthritis is another source of radial dorsal wrist pain. This joint is evaluated by instructing the patient to oppose the thumb and small finger. With ulnar deviation of the wrist, palpate just distal to the scaphoid, identifying the trapezium. Gentle thumb rotation can help differentiate between the base of the metacarpal and the trapezium. Tenderness here may indicate scaphotrapezial joint arthritis.

The thumb carpometacarpal (CMC) joint is a common source of radial dorsal zone pain. The thumb CMC joint is identified by abducting the thumb and palpating proximally along the dorsal aspect of the thumb metacarpal until a small depression is reached (Figure 2-4). This is the CMC joint. Pain here may indicate CMC arthritis.

The CMC grind test is performed by applying an axial load with rotation to the thumb metacarpal. Note the presence of crepitus and/or pain, as some patients have clinical and radiographic evidence of CMC arthritis with minimal pain.

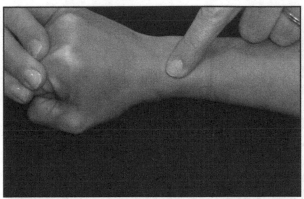

Figure 2-5. Palpation of the second dorsal extensor compartment tendons.

The thumb CMC instability test can detect ligamentous laxity and subluxation leading to pain and predisposing patients to arthritic wear. This test is performed by applying an axial distraction force to the thumb metacarpal followed by radial translation of the metacarpal base.

Tendonitis and tenosynovitis of the first 3 dorsal extensor compartments can be another source of radial dorsal wrist pain. Palpate along each tendon to evaluate for tenderness, nodules, and crepitus. The APL and EPB define the radial border of the snuffbox, and the EPL defines the ulnar border. The APL is radial to the EPB in the first dorsal compartment. The extensor carpi radialis longus (ECRL) lies radial to the extensor carpi radialis brevis (ECRB) in the second dorsal compartment (Figure 2-5). The ECRL inserts into the base of the index metacarpal, and the ECRB inserts into the base of the middle metacarpal. Pain along the course of the tendons may indicate tendonitis or tenosynovitis.

Finkelstein's test evaluates for tenosynovitis of the first dorsal compartment, commonly known as de Quervain's tenosynovitis. The thumb is flexed and held in a fist while the wrist is ulnarly deviated. Pain reproducing a patient's symptoms confirms de Quervain's tenosynovitis.

Intersection syndrome is a tenosynovitis of the second dorsal extensor compartment proximal and slightly ulnar to the site of de Quervain's. It results from friction as the APL and EPB muscle bellies cross over the ECRL and ECRB tendons.

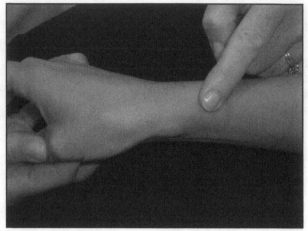

Figure 2-6. Performance of a Tinel's test over the DSRN.

Palpate 4 to 5 cm proximal to the radial styloid with active thumb motion to detect tenderness and friction.

The dorsal sensory radial nerve (DSRN) is another potential source of radial dorsal zone pain. Evaluate for hypersensitivity, sensibility, numbness, and tingling. Perform a Tinel's test by percussing along the course of the nerve (Figure 2-6). Irritation of the DSRN is called Wartenberg's syndrome. It may occur secondary to extrinsic compression or radial-sided wrist injuries. Pain is usually 1 to 2 cm proximal to the radial styloid and radiates distally over the dorsal web space and thumb. Volar ulnar wrist flexion stretches the nerve and may reproduce or exacerbate symptoms.

Central Dorsal Zone

Examination of the dorsal central zone begins with identification of Lister's tubercle. This bony prominence over the dorsal surface of the distal radius is an important landmark, often used to locate other structures. It separates the scaphoid fossa from the lunate fossa on the distal radius.

The lunate is palpated distal and ulnar to Lister's tubercle. Wrist flexion uncovers the lunate, and it forms a round prominence. Focal tenderness over the lunate may indicate Kienböck disease or lunate fracture.

The SL interval is identified slightly radial to the lunate, with the wrist flexed (Figure 2-7). Moving the wrist into radial

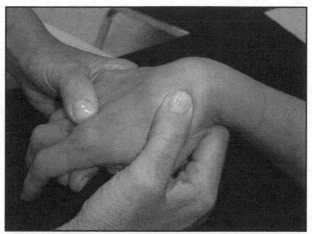

Figure 2-7. Identification of the SL interval.

and ulnar deviation helps to identify this interval, which lies between the third and fourth extensor compartments, distal and ulnar to Lister's tubercle. Assess for tenderness, widening of the interval, fullness, and clicking. These may indicate an occult dorsal wrist ganglion, SL dissociation, or rotatory subluxation of the scaphoid. Dorsal wrist syndrome presents with pain here as well and results from localized dorsal SL synovitis secondary to excessive stress on the local ligamentous structures. The finger extension test evaluates for dorsal wrist syndrome by resisting finger extension in the flexed wrist. Pain in the SL interval with this maneuver is considered a positive test.

Rotatory subluxation of the scaphoid can occur from acute or chronic SL ligament injury. Tenderness at the articular junction over the scaphoid ridge, synovitis at the triscaphe joint, dorsal SL synovitis, a positive finger extension test, and a scaphoid shift test can all point to rotatory subluxation.

The scaphoid shift test (Watson's test, radial stress test) evaluates for SL instability. Grasp the wrist from the radial side with the thumb over the volar prominence of the scaphoid and the fingers around the dorsal distal radius. Wrist position is controlled with the other hand. Apply constant thumb pressure to the scaphoid, and move the wrist from ulnar deviation and slight extension into radial deviation and flexion (Figure 2-8). In the normal wrist, the scaphoid will palmarly

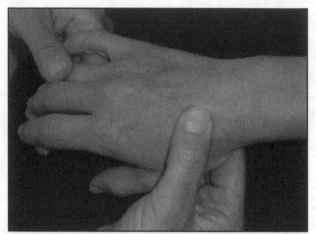

Figure 2-8. Palpation of index and middle finger CMC joints.

flex with radial deviation and push the examiner's thumb out of the way. With ligamentous laxity, the scaphoid shifts up onto the dorsal rim of the distal radius with thumb pressure and returns to its normal position with a "clunk" when thumb pressure is withdrawn. A positive test elicits a painful click or clunk that reproduces the patient's symptoms.

The scaphoid thrust test (Lane) also evaluates SL instability. A dorsally directed force is applied to the scaphoid tubercle, and a dorsal shift reproducing symptoms is considered a positive test.

Central wrist pain over the capitate is evaluated by palpating proximal to the base of middle finger metacarpal, distal to the lunate. A small depression is felt, representing the neck of the capitate. Tenderness here may be associated with SL instability, lunotriquetral (LT) instability, capitolunate arthritis, or midcarpal instability.

Pain more distally in the central dorsal zone may occur at the base of the index and middle finger metacarpals and CMC joints. Palpate proximally along the index and long metacarpals to the base, which is slightly more prominent than the shaft (see Figure 2-8). Tenderness may indicate injury to these joints, which can occur with forced palmar flexion of the wrist and hand. A metacarpal boss may be present. This bony prominence is typically found near the ECRL and ECRB

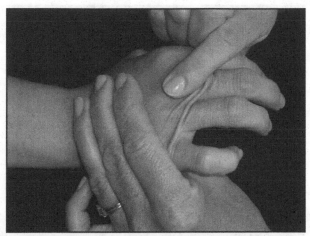

Figure 2-9. Linscheid's test for CMC ligament injury.

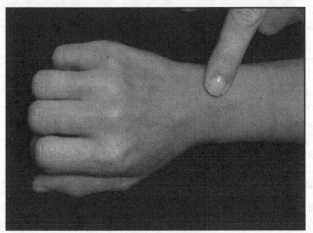

Figure 2-10. Palpation of EDC tendons.

insertions and can be caused by chronic sprains at the CMC joints. Linscheid test for CMC ligament injury is performed by supporting the metacarpal shaft and applying a palmar and dorsal stress at the metacarpal head (Figure 2-9). Subtle subluxation causing pain indicates a ligament injury.

Tendonitis and inflammation of the extensor digitorum communis (EDC) tendons may cause dorsal central wrist pain. Palpate the EDC tendons just ulnar to Lister's tubercle and note any tenderness, swelling, or crepitus (Figure 2-10). Test

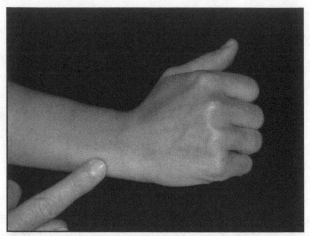

Figure 2-11. Palpation of the ulnar head.

active finger extension against resistance to detect inflammation.

The terminal end of the posterior interosseous nerve (PIN) lies deep to the fourth dorsal compartment and provides sensory innervation to the dorsal wrist capsule. This may be a source of pain when a ganglion distends the wrist capsule. Neuroma of the PIN after surgical approaches may also cause pain. Palpate proximal and ulnar to Lister's tubercle to evaluate for the PIN as a pain source.

Ulnar Dorsal Zone

Ulnar-sided wrist pain was once considered to be a "black box" filled with poorly understood causes of chronic, difficult-to-treat pathology. With increased understanding of the anatomic basis of ulnar-sided wrist pathology and improved examination techniques, causes of ulnar-sided wrist pain are now more easily diagnosed and treated.

Examination begins with identification and palpation of the ulnar head and ulnar styloid. The ulnar head forms a rounded prominence that becomes more evident in pronation (Figure 2-11). The ulnar styloid is found at the distal ulnar aspect of the ulna and is most prominent in neutral rotation. Tenderness directly over these bony prominences may indicate contusion or fracture.

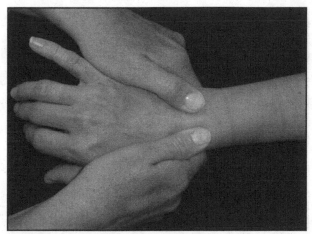

Figure 2-12. Piano key test for DRUJ instability.

The distal radioulnar joint (DRUJ) is a common source of ulnar dorsal zone pain. Palpate just radial to the ulnar head, and place one finger over the DRUJ while rotating the forearm from maximum supination to maximum pronation. Note any tenderness, abnormal volar or dorsal mobility, or change in relationship between distal radius and distal ulna. Always compare to the contralateral side.

The piano key test evaluates for DRUJ instability. Grasp the distal ulna and attempt to passively move the ulna volar and dorsal in various degrees of pronation and supination (Figure 2-12). Note any pain, tenderness, or increased mobility.

DRUJ arthritis may also cause ulnar dorsal pain and is evaluated by the DRUJ compression test. The examiner squeezes the ulnar head into the sigmoid notch of the radius in pronation (Figure 2-13). Reproduction of the patient's symptoms is considered a positive test for DRUJ arthritis. Crepitus may be appreciated with rotation and compression.

Damage to the triangular fibrocartilage complex (TFCC) is increasingly recognized as a source of ulnar dorsal wrist pain, and several examination maneuvers can be used to evaluate this structure. The TFCC can be palpated distal to the DRUJ, between the ulnar head and triquetrum. Tenderness here may indicate a TFCC problem and/or ulnocarpal abutment. Palpate the TFCC in pronation and supination. Pronation shortens the radius relative to the ulna and increases the compression

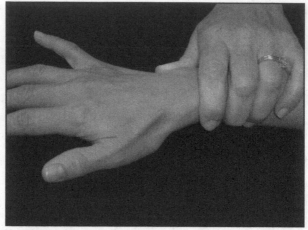

Figure 2-13. DRUJ compression test to evaluate for DRUJ arthritis.

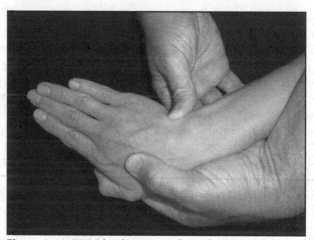

Figure 2-14. TFCC load test to evaluate for TFCC pathology and ulnocarpal abutment.

of the TFCC articular disc between the ulna and triquetrum. Ulnocarpal abutment is accentuated by pronation and ulnar deviation.

The TFCC load test is performed by flexing and extending the wrist, after application of an axial load in ulnar deviation (Figure 2-14). Pain, crepitus, and reproduction of symptoms may indicate a TFCC tear and/or ulnocarpal abutment.

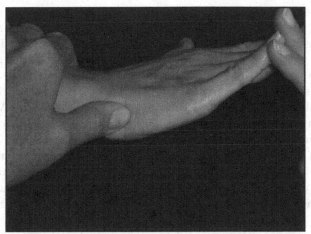

Figure 2-15. Palpation of the triquetrum in the ulnar snuff-box.

Carpal bony prominences are palpated to identify possible fractures following trauma to the wrist. The hamate is palpable just proximal to the small finger metacarpal. The triquetrum, commonly injured in a fall onto the extended wrist, is identified just distal to the ulnar styloid in the ulnar snuffbox, between the flexor carpi ulnaris (FCU) and extensor carpi ulnaris (ECU) tendons (Figure 2-15). Radial deviation of the wrist exposes the triquetrum. Tenderness at either site may indicate fracture.

Midcarpal instability may be a dorsal ulnar pain generator in patients with chronic ligamentous laxity or after a traumatic event. This entity is characterized by volar sag of the ulnar side of the wrist at rest. The midcarpal shift test evaluates for midcarpal instability. With the forearm in pronation and the wrist in neutral, apply a palmar load and axial compression to the wrist while moving from neutral to ulnar deviation. A painful clunk, reproducing the patient's symptoms, occurs with midcarpal instability.

Injury to the lunotriquetral (LT) ligament or interval is another cause of ulnar dorsal pain. This interval is palpated just ulnar to the prominence of the lunate or in line with the ring metacarpal between the EDC and EDQ tendons. Tenderness here may indicate LT injury or dissociation.

The lunotriquetral ballottement test evaluates for LT instability. The lunate is stabilized between the thumb and index of one hand, and the examiner attempts to displace the triquetrum volar and dorsal with the other hand. This test is positive with laxity, pain, crepitus, or clicking. The shuck test for LT instability is performed by placing the examiner's fingers dorsal to the lunate and thumb volar to the pisiform. Volar pressure is applied to the lunate and dorsal pressure to the pisiform, with ulnar and radial deviation of the wrist. This test is positive with pain, clicking, and reproduction of patient symptoms. The squeeze test is performed by the examiner applying a radially directed pressure to the ulnar surface of the triquetrum. This pressure accentuates the pain of LT instability.

Tendonitis or tenosynovitis on the ulnar dorsal aspect of the wrist can occur along the course of the ECU tendon. Palpate the ECU in the gap between the ulnar styloid and the small finger metacarpal in pronation and during active ulnar deviation. The ECU lies on the ulnar side of the wrist in pronation and moves dorsally over the ulnar head with supination. Tenderness may indicate tenosynovitis.

ECU subluxation may cause pain, clicking, and popping on the ulnar side of the wrist. The ECU subluxation test is performed with the forearm supinated. The patient is instructed to ulnarly deviate the wrist against resistance while the examiner palpates the ECU (Figure 2-16). Visible or palpable subluxation on the dorsal ulnar side of the wrist is a positive test. Alternatively, flexion of the wrist in this position may dislocate a subluxated tendon volarly with a palpable snap.

Radial Volar Zone

Pain in the radial volar zone may occur from fractures, arthritic conditions, tendinopathies, and compressive neuropathy. Examination begins with palpation of the scaphoid tuberosity. Radially deviate the wrist, and palpate this bony prominence at the base of the thenar crease. Tenderness here may indicate ST arthritis, distal pole scaphoid fracture, or other scaphoid pathology. The volar aspect of the radial styloid is palpated to evaluate volar radio-carpal ligament injury. Pain may be elicited with wrist extension and radial deviation.

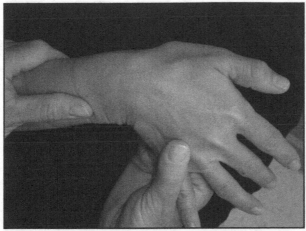

Figure 2-16. ECU subluxation test.

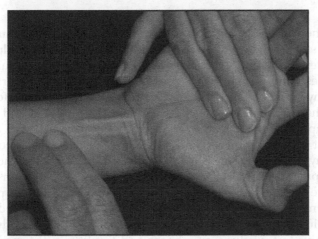

Figure 2-17. Palpation of the FCR tendon.

The thumb CMC joint can cause volar as well as dorsal radial wrist pain. Tenderness with volar palpation adjacent to the trapezial ridge may indicate thumb CMC arthritis. The CMC grind test should be performed as previously described.

The flexor carpi radialis (FCR) tendon lies radial to the palmaris longus (PL) on the volar-radial aspect of the wrist (Figure 2-17). Tenderness and swelling along the tendon and pain with resisted wrist flexion and radial deviation may indicate tenosynovitis.

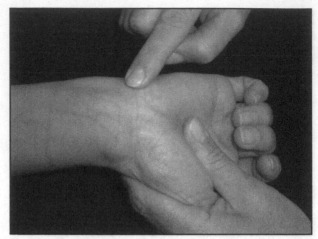

Figure 2-18. Palpation of the pisiform.

The PL tendon lies ulnar to the FCR. Oppose the thumb and small finger with wrist flexion to visualize and palpate the tendon. Eighty percent of limbs have a PL. The PL rarely causes pain, but noting its presence or absence is important in any patient being evaluated for potential tendon transfers.

The median nerve lies between and deep to FCR and PL. Compressive neuropathy is a common cause of hand and wrist pain, numbness, and tingling. The examiner should always perform Tinel's and Phalen's tests to detect nerve compression. Tinel's is performed by gently tapping over the nerve at the wrist. A positive test produces tingling and pain that may radiate to the fingers. Phalen's test is performed by holding the wrist in a flexed position for 15 to 60 seconds. A positive test produces numbness and tingling in the median nerve distribution.

Ulnar Volar Zone

Pain in the ulnar volar zone can also occur from fracture, arthritic conditions, tendinopathies, and compressive neuropathy. Bony palpation in this zone starts with the pisiform, a carpal sesamoid bone that lies within the FCU tendon. It overlies the triquetrum and is palpated at the base of the hypothenar eminence at the wrist flexion crease (Figure 2-18). When relaxed, the pisiform can be moved against the triquetrum.

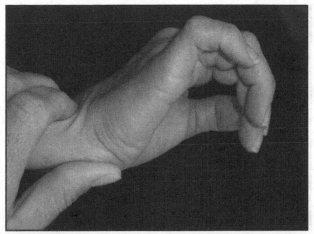

Figure 2-19. Pisiform shear test for pisotriquetral arthritis.

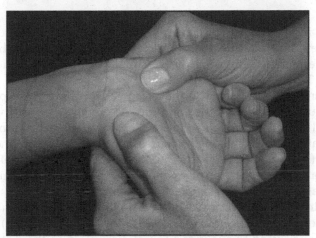

Figure 2-20. Palpation of the hook of the hamate.

The shear test is performed by applying pressure with the thumb over the pisiform and fingers dorsal to the triquetrum. The pisiform is pushed or rocked back and forth, and pain or crepitus indicates pisotriquetral arthritis (Figure 2-19).

The hook of the hamate may be an ulnar volar pain source. Fracture of this bony prominence can be seen in golfers, baseball players, and racquet sport participants. Palpate the hook of the hamate slightly radial and distal to the pisiform in the hypothenar eminence (Figure 2-20). Point tenderness here

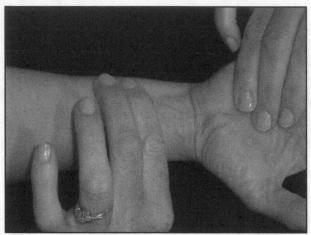

Figure 2-21. Palpation of the FCU tendon.

may indicate fracture. Patients may have associated ulnar nerve symptoms due to its intimate relationship with the hook of the hamate. The ulnar nerve should always be evaluated with Tinel's test in Guyon's canal.

Tendonitis of the FCU may also cause ulnar volar pain. Instruct the patient to flex and ulnarly deviate the wrist with small finger abduction to make the FCU tendon prominent. Palpate the tendon along its course, and note any focal tenderness (Figure 2-21). It inserts into the pisiform, the hook of the hamate through the pisohamate ligament, and the fifth metacarpal through the pisometacarpal ligament.

Ulnar volar pain can also be related to TFCC and/or ulnotriquetral ligament injury. The ulnar fovea sign (Berger's) is a maneuver used to evaluate a foveal disruption in these structures. The examiner presses firmly into the interval between the ulnar styloid and FCU or the volar surface of the ulnar styloid and pisiform (Figure 2-22). This test is considered positive when the patient's pain is reproduced.

GENERAL TESTS

Some additional maneuvers can detect more generalized problems or pathology that involves multiple zones. Allen's

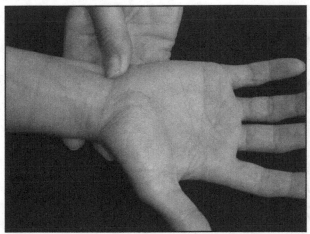

Figure 2-22. Ulnar foveal palpation (Berger's sign) for TFCC or ulnotriquetral ligament injury.

test evaluates patency of the radial and ulnar arteries and should be a part of every wrist exam. The patient is instructed to open and close the hand several times forcefully and then hold a tight fist while the examiner occludes both the radial and ulnar arteries. The examiner then releases the radial artery and observes for flushing. The test is then repeated to test the ulnar artery. If the patient's skin stays white and blanched, there may be an occlusion.

The carpal shake test is performed to detect and assess the presence of synovitis. The examiner grasps the distal forearm and shakes or passively flexes and extends the wrist (Figure 2-23). This will be painful in the presence of significant synovitis.

The sitting hands test may also detect synovitis and may indicate scapholunate ligament injury. Ask the patient to place both hands on the seat of a chair and push off (Figure 2-24). This will be too difficult and painful for a patient with significant synovitis or SL ligament injury.

Finally, grip testing can be a reliable indicator of a pathologic process that warrants further investigation in cases of obscure wrist pain. Lister and colleagues found a significant correlation between decreased grip strength and positive bone scans with confirmed pathology in patients with chronic

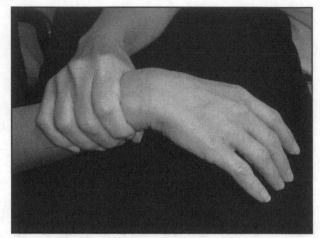

Figure 2-23. Carpal shake test to evaluate for synovitis.

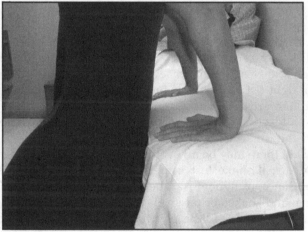

Figure 2-24. Sitting hands or push-off test will produce pain in a patient with synovitis or SL ligament injury.

wrist complaints. Submaximal effort was ruled out with rapid exchange grip testing and a bell-shaped curve with five-position grip testing.

CONCLUSION

Using these techniques, a skilled clinician can obtain a thorough and accurate patient history and perform a well-executed wrist examination to form an accurate differential diagnosis. Further imaging and electro-diagnostic studies can then be used to confirm diagnoses and direct appropriate treatment for painful wrist conditions.

SUGGESTED READING

Cooney WP, Linscheid RL, Dobyns JH. *The wrist: Diagnosis and operative treatment*. St. Louis, MO: Mosby; 1998:236-261.

Gilula LA, Yin Y. *Imaging of the wrist and hand*. Philadelphia: W.B. Saunders Co; 1996:5-18, 23-42.

Kleinman WB. Stability of the distal radioulnar joint: biomechanics, pathophysiology, physical diagnosis, and restoration of function. What we have learned in 25 years. *J Hand Surg*. 2007;32A:1086-1106.

Lichtman DM, Alexander AH. *The wrist and its disorders*. Philadelphia: W.B. Saunders; 1997:73-90.

Skirven TM, Osterman AL. *Clinical examination of the wrist in rehabilitation of the hand and upper extremity*. St. Louis, MO: Mosby; 2002:1099-1116.

Taleisnik J. *The wrist*. New York: Churchill Livingston; 1985:1-38.

Tay SC, Tomita K, Berger RA. The "ulnar foveal sign" for defining ulnar wrist pain: an analysis of sensitivity and specificity. *J Hand Surg*. 2007;32A:438-444.

Whipple TL. *Arthroscopic surgery: The wrist*. Philadelphia: J.B. Lippincott Co; 1992:11-36.

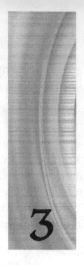

3

PHYSICAL
EXAMINATION
OF THE HAND
THE BASICS AND SPECIFIC TESTS

John J. Fernandez, MD, FAAOS

INTRODUCTION

An efficient and thorough physical examination of the hand can be challenging. This is particularly true if the hand is in pain or has been recently injured. A working knowledge of pertinent anatomy is fundamental. Understanding biomechanical function and relative anatomic relationships is essential to understanding normal function and ultimately recognizing pathology.

Culp RW, Jacoby SM. *Musculoskeletal Examination of the Elbow, Wrist, and Hand: Making the Complex Simple* (pp. 36-71). © 2012 Taylor & Francis Group.

Table 3-1

PRIOR HISTORY

- Injuries
- Surgeries
- Medical conditions
- Tobacco, alcohol, and other drug use
- Hobbies, recreational activities, occupation
- Mechanism of injury
- Loss of function

Table 3-2

SYMPTOMS

- Location
- Type
- Intensity
- Frequency
- Alleviating/aggravating factors

The patient history is crucial and can be considered the "preface" of the physical examination. This includes eliciting presenting complaints as well as any prior history. The prior history should encompass previous injuries, surgeries, associated medical conditions, and all prior treatment leading up to the examination (Table 3-1).

The presenting complaints begin with a description of "when" and "how" the problem began and what has been done to date. If the problem was traumatic in origin, the mechanism of injury should be detailed (ie, forces involved, position of joints).

The patient's symptoms are detailed as to their location, type, intensity, duration, and frequency. Any associated, aggravating, and/or alleviating factors should also be searched for in the history (Table 3-2).

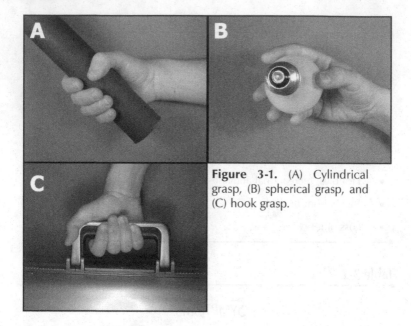

Figure 3-1. (A) Cylindrical grasp, (B) spherical grasp, and (C) hook grasp.

Finally, the exam should focus on the patient's perception of his or her dysfunction (loss of function). Hand function is a complex interplay between all of the digits and/or the palm. It primarily depends on the ability to "grip." Grip function can be categorized as power grip and precision grip. Power grip includes cylindrical, spherical, and hook grasp (Figure 3-1). Precision grip includes pulp pinch, lateral (key) pinch, and chuck pinch (Figure 3-2). Understanding these functions and whether they are affected in the patient is very helpful.

While much of this information can be obtained verbally, it is preferable to also have the patient document it in the form of a questionnaire. This would include a pain diagram and visual analogue scale.

After the history is obtained, 2 types of physical examination can be performed: problem oriented or systematic. A problem-oriented examination focuses on the areas that are affected. While this approach to the physical examination is efficient, it can overlook subtle or related findings. This can result in a faulty diagnosis or "missed" diagnosis of associated injuries or conditions. A "systematic" approach involves a comprehensive examination of the hand regardless of the

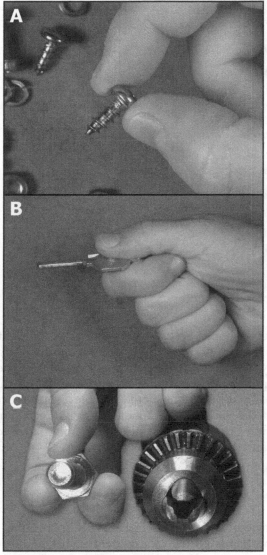

Figure 3-2. (A) Pulp (tip; precision) pinch, (B) lateral (key) pinch, and (C) chuck pinch.

complaint. This approach can avoid the pitfalls of the problem-oriented exam and is therefore recommended.

The examination of the hands should be performed with the patient and examiner comfortably seated and facing each

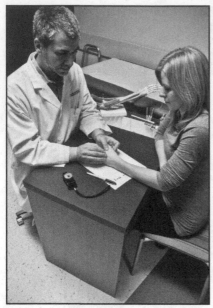

Figure 3-3. Patient seated comfortably across from examiner with hands supported and tools nearby.

other. There should be a waist-height table or platform on which to rest the elbow and forearm during the examination, preferably with comfortable padding (Figure 3-3). The examination equipment should be nearby to maintain a rhythm to the exam. This equipment should include a soft tape measure, two-point discriminator, goniometer, grip meter, and pinch meter. The examiner should also have note paper to record findings and draw figures if needed (Figure 3-4).

INSPECTION

The physical examination begins with inspection, and not just of the hand but also the patient in his or her entirety. Observations are made of the patient's mannerisms, behavior, and his or her interactions and reactions to the examiner as well as the exam itself. During the exam, the patient's effort and consistency of complaints are judged.

Both hands are visually inspected simultaneously making comparisons between both sides. The inspection is performed

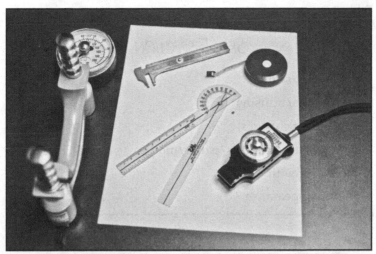

Figure 3-4. Tape measure, two-point discriminator, goniometer, grip meter, pinch meter, and note paper.

while the digits are held in full extension, full flexion, and during the process of active extension and flexion. Begin with the patient holding both hands palm up (supinated), and then have him or her pronate palm down to finish inspecting the dorsal hand.

Examine the skin for any lesions or scars (Table 3-3). If there has been recent trauma, wounds or bruising are noted and described. Measurements are made for length, width, depth, and location using relative topographical landmarks such as skin creases.

Skin color is determined by a combination of skin thickness, pigment, and vascularity. Note if there are any circumscribed areas of atrophy, thinning, or changes in pigmentation. Vascular anomalies can affect skin color through increased venous congestion, decreased arterial perfusion, or a combination of the 2, creating cyanosis, pallor, or mottling. Try to differentiate certain types of color changes such as erythema, which may be indicative of an infection, versus the normal reactive healing process. Inspect the hair and nails, and note changes such as increased or decreased growth, thickening or thinning, and brittleness (Figure 3-5).

Table 3-3

SKIN INSPECTION

- Lesions/scars
- Wounds/bruising
- Pigment changes
- Erythema/cyanosis/pallor/mottling
- Hair growth
- Nail appearance

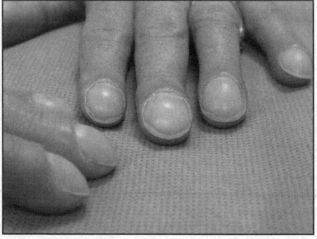

Figure 3-5. Nail appearance, such as clubbing (shown here), can be an indication of underlying systemic pathology.

Any deformity is assessed in comparison to the contralateral side. Deformity can be caused by abnormalities of the soft tissues, tumors, and changes in normal alignment (Table 3-4). The soft tissues can contribute through local and generalized edema, thickening of the ligaments or tendons, and atrophy of the muscles. Tumors can create a local mass effect from a cystic

Table 3-4

CAUSES OF DEFORMITY

- Edema
- Tumors
- Fracture malunions
- Dislocations
- Arthritis (osteoarthritis, rheumatoid)
- Instability (ligament injury, lupus)

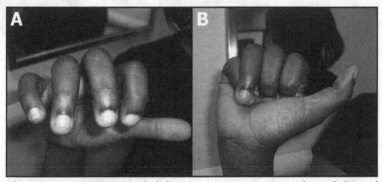

Figure 3-6. (A) Rotational deformity in extension may be subtle and unnoticed. (B) Rotational deformity in flexion is usually magnified.

or solid mass. Changes in alignment can result from fracture malunions and instability or laxity of the joints.

It is important to assess deformity with the digits in both full extension and flexion, as in some cases the deformity is dynamic and will change severity with position. This is particularly true with fracture malunions in the hand and digits (Figure 3-6). Position of the wrist can affect the appearance and alignment of the digits. If there is angular or rotational deformity, describe its location, severity, and what plane it occupies.

Certain "named" deformities have a characteristic appearance and can give important clues regarding underlying

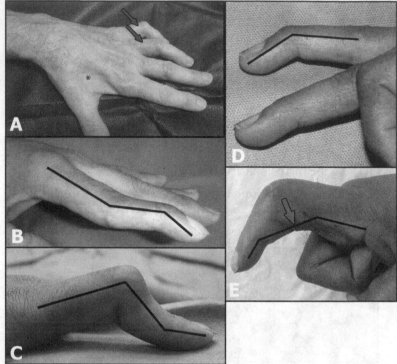

Figure 3-7. (A) Claw hand as a result of ulnar neuropathy. Note relative extension through metacarpophalangeal joints and flexion through interphalangeal joints affecting ring and small fingers more severely (arrows). There is also atrophy of first dorsal interosseous muscle (asterisk). (B) Swan-neck deformity with hyperextension at proximal interphalangeal joint and flexion at distal interphalangeal joint secondary to volar plate insufficiency and tendon imbalance. (C) Boutonnière deformity with flexion at proximal interphalangeal joint and extension at distal interphalangeal joint secondary to central slip insufficiency. (D) Mallet deformity with flexion deformity at distal interphalangeal joint secondary to terminal tendon insufficiency. (E) Bowstringing deformity from palmar subluxation of flexor tendons secondary to incompetent pulley system. Flexion contracture can ensue.

pathology. These include claw hand, swan-neck, boutonnière, mallet, and bowstringing deformities (Figure 3-7).

Local edema or thickening is recorded with circumferential measurements at different locations such as the wrist, midpalm, and individual joints and phalanges (Figure 3-8). This method is rapid and simple to perform. It is most effective in

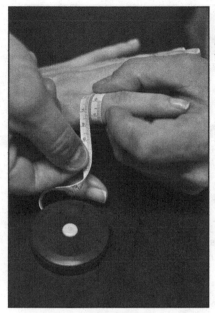

Figure 3-8. Circumferential measurements can be taken at any level and compared against the contralateral side.

assessing local findings but is less precise with generalized edema. Generalized edema is more precisely measured with volumetric techniques. This is done by immersing the hand up to the wrist into a container of water and then measuring the amount of water displaced. Quantifying edema can be helpful when trying to assess the hand over time.

Atrophy of the muscles can sometimes be difficult to appreciate and quantify, especially if there is concurrent edema or deformity. It is best appreciated in the thenar muscles at the base of the thumb and the first dorsal interosseous and adductor muscles of the first dorsal webspace (Figure 3-9).

The inspection process does not begin and end by itself. It continues during other portions of the examination and should be used to detect findings such as triggering or locking of joints, subluxation of tendons, and tendon adhesions to skin or scar.

PALPATION

While the palpation portion of the examination is used primarily in addressing areas of pain or masses, it also can

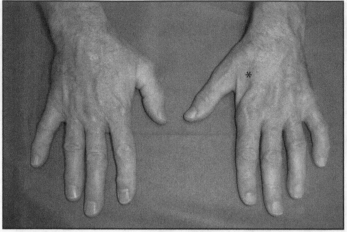

Figure 3-9. Atrophy of intrinsic muscles secondary to ulnar neuropathy. First doral interosseous muscle atrophy noted with asterisk.

provide other important information. This process is more problem or complaint oriented. It is still vital to examine the other hand for comparison. Some patients can have "normal" complaints of discomfort or unusual findings, and it is important to distinguish this from actual pathology.

The skin is addressed first and is assessed for temperature, sweat pattern, and vascularity. With both of the patient's hands held palm-up, the examiner can use the dorsum of his or her own hands to quickly distinguish if there are temperature differences from one side to the other. Differences in sweat pattern can also be felt while touching and wiping the tips of the digits.

This is a good point to assess capillary refill. Gentle pressure is applied to the pulp of the fingertips with the tip of a pen to blanch them of color. The color of the nail beds while pinching the fingertip can be used as a marker, but this is usually more uncomfortable and less reliable. The time needed for the color to return is noted and compared to the contralateral side and within the same hand. Normal capillary refill occurs within 2 to 3 seconds. If there is venous congestion, capillary refill can be false-normal. In these cases, the hands should be elevated above the level of the heart and then retested.

Masses are noted for their location, size, and consistency. The patient should be asked to move his or her digits to see if the mass moves with the tendons, implying their origin. In some cases, the tendons can pass over the mass, creating mechanical symptoms such as clicking or snapping.

If pain is a primary complaint, have the patient point to or circle the area that he or she perceives as the source. If symptoms seem generalized or referred from other areas, try to have the patient localize the origin. If there are multiple areas, have the patient "rank" them in order of severity. Before palpating the area of pain, it is useful to begin on the contralateral hand so the patient knows what to expect. It is also helpful to tell him or her that you will begin with a gentle amount of pressure.

The anatomically compact nature of the hand can make it difficult to distinguish which structures may be generating pain (ie, joint, ligament, or tendon). The examiner should try isolating these structures so that they are assessed individually. The very tip of the index finger or small finger should be used to palpate as the pulp itself tends to exert a diffuse and imprecise area of pressure. This can lead to a false impression of the origin of tenderness.

Pain elicited during the exam can be difficult to judge, as it is subjective by its very nature. Using a numeric analogue scale from 1 to 10 is helpful, particularly if there are multiple areas causing pain. It is also helpful to contrast multiple areas of pain in close proximity. For example, ask, "Which hurts more, point A or point B?" By moving back and forth, the examiner can gain a better understanding of the maximum point of tenderness and discern its possible source.

Palpation of the joints can result in pain originating from the joint itself, its ligaments, or the tendons that cross it. While joint pain can be elicited by pressure from any direction, it is more difficult to elicit from the palmar region because of the thickness of the flexor tendons and volar plates. If there is tenderness along the palmar region, it can be related to the flexor tendons or volar plate.

The joints are most exposed along their dorsoradial and dorsoulnar surfaces where there are no ligaments or tendons to shield them. The ligaments are exposed along the lateral joint surfaces. When applying pressure from the sides, such as "squeezing" a joint, it should be noted which side is the one generating the pain. This can indicate pathology of the joint, the ligament, or both. Note if there is any triggering, locking, or crepitus of the joint or tendon with motion of the digit.

Specifically, palpate the insertion sites of the tendons and ligaments to help differentiate those as a source of joint pain. By having the patient actively resist extension or flexion of the digits, increased pain can be attributed to a tendon origin. By comparison, pain that remains static, regardless of applied resistance, can be an indication of joint origin.

Stability of the joint depends on both bony and soft tissue constraints. This varies depending upon the joint. The metacarpophalangeal joints rely more heavily on the soft tissue envelope (ie, collateral ligaments, volar plate, and capsule). The interphalangeal joints by comparison rely more equally on the soft tissues as well as the bony constraints of the joint.

The collateral ligaments are assessed by stressing them in the radial and ulnar direction with the joints held in various positions of extension and flexion. The findings and their significance can vary widely, depending on the joint and digit, and must be compared bilaterally.

The metacarpophalangeal joints have a unique design in that the metacarpal head is ovoid in shape and increases in width from dorsal to palmar. This property gives the joint increased mobility at the expense of stability while in extension. With increasing flexion, the ligament has a "cam effect" in which it comes under increasing tension. When examining these ligaments, the joint must be held in maximum allowable flexion (Figure 3-10). The amount of allowable flexion usually increases from the index to the small finger and is typically a minimum of 90 degrees. There is also a small amount of rotation that can be elicited through the joint while traveling in its arc of motion. It can be difficult in the nonborder digits, as the adjacent digits can block the examination.

Thumb metacarpophalangeal joint motion exhibits the most "normal" variability among individuals. It can flex as little as 10 degrees or 20 degrees, up to more than 90 degrees. The thumb metacarpal collateral ligaments are stressed with the joint in 30 degrees of flexion (Figure 3-11). Comparisons are made from side to side, as there can be a wide range of normal.[1]

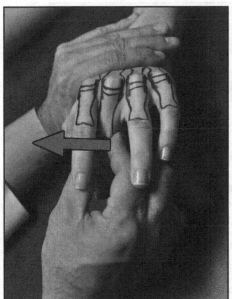

Figure 3-10. Metacarpophalangeal ligament examination is performed with the joint in near full flexion with the other digits in slight extension. Stress is being applied across the middle finger toward the index finger, testing the ulnar collateral ligament.

Hyperextension in the joints can be a normal finding, particularly in the ring and small finger but can also be abnormal secondary to insufficiency of the volar plate. This can be particularly problematic in the thumb. Bilateral comparisons must be made and painful dysfunction documented.

The interphalangeal joints are relatively stable in all positions in comparison to the increasing stability in flexion exhibited by the metacarpophalangeal joints. These joints are stabilized in the coronal plane by the collateral ligaments. The extensor mechanism and volar plate provide stability in the sagittal plane. There can be individual variability in hyperextension through the proximal interphalangeal joint. This can also be abnormal and can lead to conditions such as swan-neck deformity.

The carpometacarpal joints also exhibit variability depending on the digit. The thumb carpometacarpal joint is saddle-shaped and exhibits the most motion. It can move in flexion-extension, adduction-abduction, and some rotation. This multi-planar movement gives the thumb its unique property of opposition. Like the interphalangeal joint, stability of

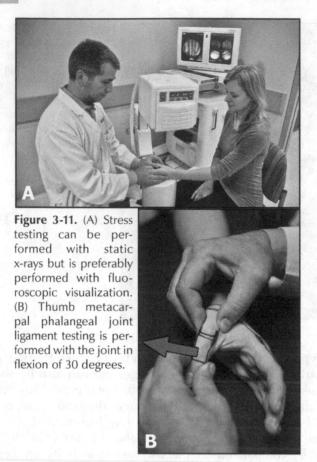

Figure 3-11. (A) Stress testing can be performed with static x-rays but is preferably performed with fluoroscopic visualization. (B) Thumb metacarpal phalangeal joint ligament testing is performed with the joint in flexion of 30 degrees.

the carpometacarpal joint depends on both bone and soft-tissue constraints. Stability is primarily assessed in the dorsal palmar plane and can be stressed with or without load placed across the joint (Figure 3-12). This is referred to as a "shuck test" or "grind test." The distal end of the thumb metacarpal is grasped with the examiner's index finger and thumb dorsal and palmar. Stress is then applied in the dorsal palmar plane while pulling and pushing across the joint.

The carpometacarpal joints of the index and middle fingers are relatively immobile, exhibiting minor amounts of extension-flexion in the sagittal plane. Any significant motion in these joints, particularly if associated with pain, should

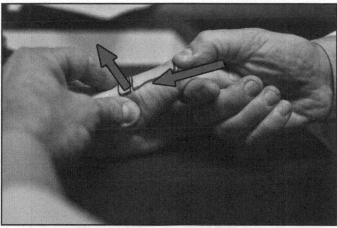

Figure 3-12. Thumb carpometacarpal joint shuck test is performed with application of axial load and translating joint dorsal and volar.

cause suspicion and be more carefully evaluated. Linscheid's test is performed by supporting the hand and pushing over the second and third metacarpal heads palmarly (Figure 3-13). Pain localized to those carpometacarpal joints is considered a positive test indicative of pathology in those joints.

By comparison, the ring and small finger carpometacarpal joints have more motion and the ability to translate and rotate. Similar to the thumb, these joints can be "shucked" in the dorsal palmar plane to assess stability.

While stress testing any of the ligaments, observations are made on whether pain is elicited and whether the ligament reaches an endpoint. Ligament injuries and laxity can be graded 1, 2, or 3. Grade 1 injuries present with pain but no laxity. Grade 2 injuries have laxity compared to the contralateral side but with an endpoint. Grade 3 injuries have gross instability without an endpoint (Table 3-5).

SURFACE ANATOMY

It is important to understand the relationship between the surface topography of the hand and its deeper structures. This is one of the cornerstones to the examination itself.

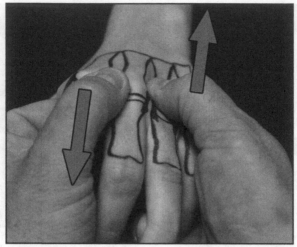

Figure 3-13. Linsheid's test is performed by stabilizing the ulnar hand and radial hand while extending and flexing at the carpometacarpal joint.

Table 3-5

LIGAMENT STABILITY

Grade 1—Pain without laxity

Grade 2—Laxity with endpoint

Grade 3—Laxity without endpoint

The dorsal and palmar skin creases serve as excellent landmarks of the relative positions of the tendons, nerves, and joints (Figure 3-14). Abnormal findings, such as masses or areas of pain, can be referenced to these landmarks.

RANGE OF MOTION

There are several measurements that can be recorded when assessing range of motion. Active motion is first measured

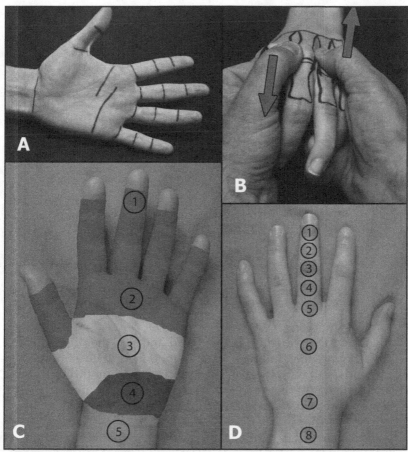

Figure 3-14. (A/B) Skin creases can be used to approximate deeper anatomy. Shown are the wrist flexion crease, distal palmar crease, and digital creases. (C) Flexor tendon zones 1 through 5 from distal to proximal. Zone 1 extends to distal A4 pulley, zone 2 extends to proximal A1 pulley, zone 3 extends to distal carpal tunnel ligament, zone 4 is the area under the carpal tunnel ligament, and zone 5 is proximal to carpal tunnel ligament. (D) Extensor tendon zones 1 through 8. Odd numbered zones correspond to areas over joints. Even number zones are areas between joints.

Figure 3-15. Goniometric measurement of digit.

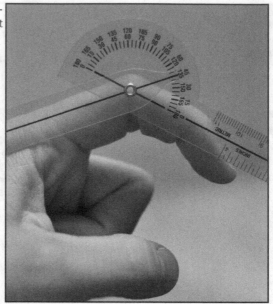

by asking the patient to fully extend and flex the digits and then noting the findings. Passive motion is then similarly measured but with the examiner placing the digit through its arc of motion. If there is a loss in active or passive motion, the reason is recorded (ie, limited by pain, weakness, stiffness, or physical block).

Each particular joint can be measured separately (Figure 3-15). In cases where there is a loss in motion at several joint levels, a "composite" measurement can be recorded as "total active motion" by adding the numbers together (Figure 3-16). If multiple digits and joints have been affected, an estimate of composite flexion can be made by measuring a "tip-to-palm" distance between the tip of the digit and the palmar surface of the hand. This is particularly helpful when assessing a patient over time for improvements in flexion, especially when multiple digits or joints are involved.

The carpometacarpal joint of the thumb can be difficult to measure because of its multiplanar movement. One plane is measured as radial abduction (extension) by measuring the thumb web-space while the hand is flat (Figure 3-17). This can

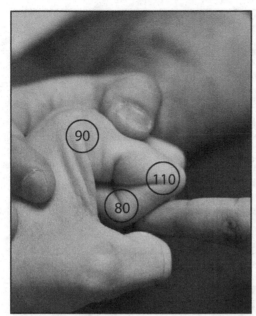

Figure 3-16. Total active motion is the sum of the figures from each joint level. In this example, 90 + 110 + 80, or 280 degrees of total active motion (TAM).

be measured as an angle or distance. The other is measured as palmar abduction (flexion) or opposition and is measured as the distance from the distal flexion crease of the thumb to the distal palmar crease of the middle finger.

It is helpful to have a printed diagram of the hand that allows for recording these measurements at their respective levels. Even tracing the hand on a paper can serve this purpose. The convention is to record the numbers similar to a "fraction" with the top number denoting extension and the bottom number denoting flexion. If there is hyperextension in a joint, the plus sign is placed in front of the number. A minus sign should not be used to note a loss of motion. Instead, the maximum number achieved should be recorded.

A disparity between joint active and passive motion should be noted as an "active-passive mismatch" and the difference recorded. This can be the result of tendon adhesions or pain that functionally limits active motion (Figure 3-18). If there is an active-passive mismatch, the passive motion measurements are written next to the active measurements but are placed in parentheses.

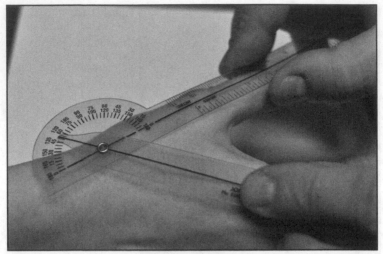

Figure 3-17. Thumb webspace measurement.

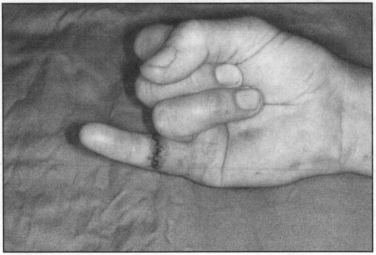

Figure 3-18. Active-passive mismatch with hand attempting flexion, noting inability to flex the small finger while being able to passively flex the digit.

Because the tendons that move the digits cross several joints, range of motion in a joint can be affected by joints proximally, including the wrist. This is particularly evident with the extensor tendons. If a loss in digit flexion is noted, then the

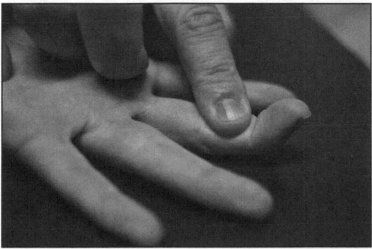

Figure 3-19. Flexor profundus testing performed by blocking the digit short of the distal interphalangeal joint while allowing the adjacent digits to flex freely.

joint must be tested with the proximal joints in varying positions of full extension and flexion. This can help distinguish whether the loss in motion is within the joint itself or related to the tendons crossing the joint.

The profundus tendons are tested individually by blocking the digit proximally at the level of the metacarpophalangeal joint and proximal interphalangeal joint (Figure 3-19). The superficialis tendons are tested while neutralizing the adjacent digits by maintaining them in full extension (Figure 3-20).

The Bunnell-Littler (intrinsic-plus) test is performed by attempting to flex the proximal interphalangeal joint while holding the metacarpal joint in either full extension or full flexion. If flexion at the interphalangeal joint worsens with increasing metacarpal extension (claw position), this is an indication of "intrinsic tightness" (Figure 3-21). This usually originates from pathology within the hand, such as fibrosis of the intrinsic muscles or tendons. If there is no change in motion at the interphalangeal joint regardless of the position of the metacarpal joint, then the pathology is likely within the joint itself or the capsule and tendons around the joint causing a fixed contracture.

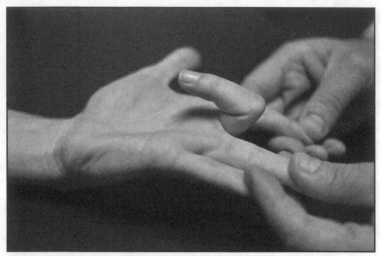

Figure 3-20. Flexor superficialis testing performed by holding the adjacent digits in extension while allowing the digit being tested to flex.

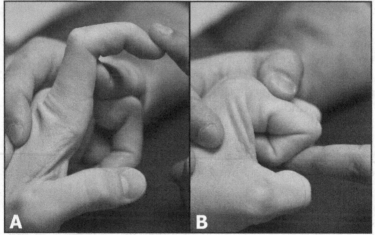

Figure 3-21. (A) Intrinsic tightness demonstrated by decreased ability to flex at distal joints while metacarpal joint is in extension. (B) Intrinsic tightness is relieved with metacarpal joint flexion, which allows the distal joints to flex.

Similarly, the motion at the metacarpophalangeal and interphalangeal joints can be affected by positions of the wrist. If flexion is limited at the distal joints with the wrist in increasing flexion, this can be a sign of "extrinsic tightness"

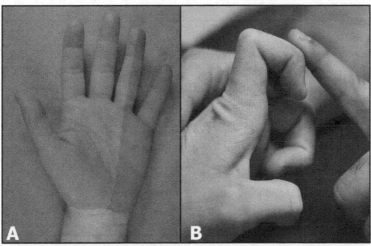

Figure 3-22. (A) Extrinsic tightness demonstrated by decreased ability to flex at distal joints while metacarpal joint is in flexion. (B) Extrinsic tightness is relieved with metacarpal joint extension, which allows the distal joints to flex.

(Figure 3-22). This usually involves extensor tendon adhesions or shortening of the tendons at the wrist or dorsal hand.

Like other parts of the body, there is variability within the hand from patient to patient. Once again, this is why it is important to use the contralateral hand as a source of what is normal for that particular patient. If both hands are affected in a similar fashion, then normative data can be used for comparison (Table 3-6).

STRENGTH TESTING

The information gained from strength testing can be used to assess neurologic function and help gauge functional capacity in the upper extremity.

Strength testing is broken down into gross neuromuscular testing or metric grip-and-pinch strength testing. Neuromuscular testing can be used to appraise individual muscles, but more commonly tests major muscle groups and the nerves that serve them. Grip-and-pinch strength is a

Table 3-6

RANGE OF MOTION

DIGITS

Metacarpophalangeal joint: +10 to 100

Proximal interphalangeal joint: 0 to 110

Distal interphalangeal joint: 0 to 80

THUMB

Metacarpophalangeal joint (variable): +10 to 30 to 100

Interphalangeal joint: +20 to 80

Table 3-7

STRENGTH TESTING

Grade 0—No contraction

Grade 1—Contraction without motion

Grade 2—Motion without gravity

Grade 3—Motion against gravity

Grade 4—Strength against resistence

Grade 5—Normal strength

function of overall conditioning and the composite function of several muscle groups.

Muscle strength is most commonly graded using the system proposed by the Medical Research Council of Britain (Table 3-7).[2] Grade 0 is no perceived muscle function. Grade 1 is muscle contraction but without joint motion. Grade 2 is muscle contraction with joint motion but with gravity eliminated. Grade 3 is joint motion against gravity but without resistance. Grade 4 is joint motion with some resistance. Grade 5 is normal muscle strength. One of the weaknesses of this

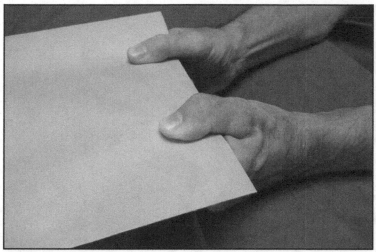

Figure 3-23. Froment's sign demonstrated by flexion through the interphalangeal joint and extension at the metacarpophalangeal joint. Comparisons can be made side to side.

grading system is the wide gap in possible function that can be seen between grade 5 and grade 3 strength. Some have suggested using pluses and minuses to further delineate those grades.

Major muscle groups are tested first, and if abnormalities are noted, then further individual testing can be performed. Begin testing with the ulnar innervated groups. Examine the ulnar intrinsics of the thumb first. Have the patient key-pinch a piece of paper while the examiner tries to pull the paper from the patient. The examiner can palpate the first dorsal interosseous muscle in the thumb webspace and observe for weakness compared to the contralateral side. If there is significant weakness, the thumb will compensate with the flexor pollicis longus and will create a hyperflexion deformity at the interphalangeal joint known as Froment's sign (Figure 3-23). The examiner can then test the intrinsic muscles of the fingers by having the patient abduct and adduct the fingers against resistance (Figure 3-24). You can also assess this by having the patient cross his or her fingers (Figure 3-25). The ulnar innervated "extrinsics" can then be tested by judging the flexor carpi ulnaris and flexor digitorum profundus muscles of the ring and small fingers. Have the patient flex his or her

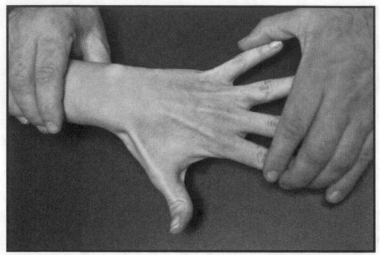

Figure 3-24. Abduction/adduction of the digits. Strength can be assessed through resisted abduction of the digits.

Figure 3-25. Cross-finger test.

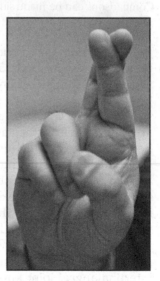

wrist against resistance, and palpate the flexor carpi ulnaris. Ask the patient to make a tight fist with the examiner pulling against the ring and small fingers.

By testing both the intrinsic and extrinsic ulnar-innervated muscles, the level of injury can be determined. Ulnar nerve

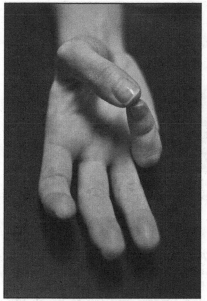

Figure 3-26. Abduction pinch.

injuries can create a characteristic "claw-hand" deformity. The metacarpophalangeal joints are held in relative extension, and the interphalangeal joints are held in flexion. The clawing is usually more severe in the ring and small fingers because the lumbricals of the index and middle fingers are preserved and contribute to intrinsic function.

High ulnar nerve injuries, at or above the level of the elbow, present with weakness of the flexor carpi ulnaris and ulnar profundus tendons. Because the profundus tendons are weakened, the claw-hand deformity can be subtle and diminished compared to low ulnar nerve injuries below the level of the elbow.

The muscles innervated by the median nerve are similarly examined as intrinsic and extrinsic muscle groups. Have the patient pinch his or her thumb tightly against the small finger while the examiner tries to break the pinch (Figure 3-26). At the same time, the thenar muscle is palpated. Atrophy and weakness are compared to the other side. The patient is asked to precision pinch the thumb and index finger together against resistance. This is also known as the "okay" sign (Figure 3-27).

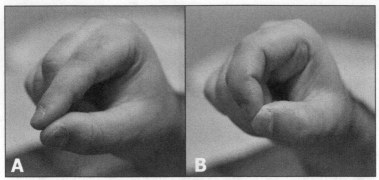

Figure 3-27. (A) Normal flexion at distal interphalangeal joints of thumb and index finger. (B) Loss of flexion at interphalangeal joints demonstrates the "okay" sign.

Inability to create or hold this position is a sign of anterior interosseous nerve dysfunction or high median nerve lesion. Have the patient curl his or her fingers into the palm around the examiner's similarly curled fingers and try to break the grasp. Weakness here can also indicate a high median nerve lesion affecting the extrinsic flexor tendons.

The radial nerve innervated muscle groups are then tested. The patient is asked to fully extend the wrist against resistance, and observations are made if there is any excess radial deviation. Weakness with radial deviation can indicate a posterior interosseous nerve lesion in contrast to a high radial nerve lesion as the radial wrist extensors are commonly innervated from the radial nerve itself. With the patient's hand flat on the table, have him or her extend the thumb toward the ceiling. This maneuver is called "retropulsion" and is impossible without normal radial nerve function (Figure 3-28). The thumb can also be tested by resisting extension at the interphalangeal joint, but it should be noted the intrinsic muscles of the thumb also contribute to extension at this level. Now, have the patient extend his or her digits against resistance at the metacarpal joints while maintaining the interphalangeal joints flexed. This is referred to as the intrinsic minus or claw-hand position (Figure 3-29). This isolates the radial nerve-innervated muscles and eliminates any contribution from the

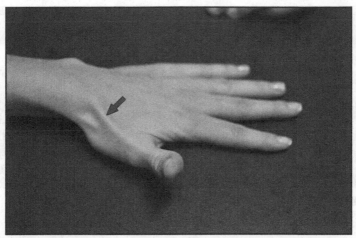

Figure 3-28. Thumb retropulsion shown by having hand flat on table and thumb extended toward ceiling. The tendon can be seen in relief.

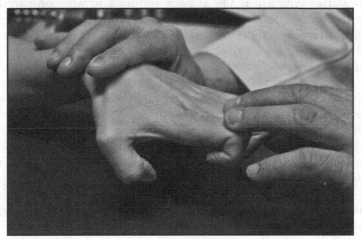

Figure 3-29. Claw extension against resistance.

intrinsic muscles, which can give a false impression of finger extension, albeit weak.

Composite strength can be tested using devices such as a Jamar dynamometer (Asimow Engineering Co, Santa Monica, CA) (Figure 3-30). This device uses an adjustable handle that can be set to 5 positions of increasing span. The handle is

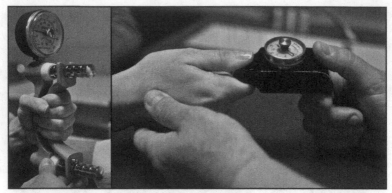

Figure 3-30. Grip   **Figure 3-31.** Pinch meter.
meter.

squeezed while using cylindrical grasp. The forces are measured in pounds or kilograms per square inch. Static strength
measurements are made at each setting and are compared
to the contralateral side. Most individuals are approximately
20% stronger on their dominant side. The measurements usually approximate a bell-shaped curve. They are usually maximal at the second position depending on the size of the hand.[3]

This test can also be performed while rapidly exchanging
from one side to the other or rapidly measuring both sides
simultaneously (rapid exchange grip).[4,5] Another variant of
this test is to have the patient repeatedly grip at a fast rate.[6]
There should be a "drop" in force when compared to static
testing. If the forces increase or stay the same, this can be a
sign of malingering or poor effort.

Pinch strength can be similarly measured with a "pinch
meter" while having the individual engage in lateral (key)
pinch or pulp pinch (Figure 3-31).

While comparisons in strength can be made from side to
side, there are also normative data that can be used depending
on age and gender.[7]

SENSORY TESTING

Sensation provides information on temperature, light and
deep touch, pressure, vibration, and pain. The perception
of sensory input is provided by mechanoreceptors. These

receptors have unique properties, which supply information to the brain. The nerve fibers themselves have distinct properties that provide sensory information and can be considered either "slowly" or "quickly" adapting nerve fibers. Slowly adapting fibers continue to respond throughout the stimulus, and their response is proportional to the stimulus. Quickly adapting fibers respond only briefly to stimulus and do not have a dose-dependent response to a stimulus.

The innervation of the hand tends to follow a relatively reproducible pattern. There can be some variability and overlap between different nerves, making an accurate diagnosis challenging or confusing.

The median nerve primarily supplies the thumb, index, middle, and the radial half of the ring finger. This includes the palmar and dorsal skin from the tips to the level of the proximal interphalangeal joints and the palmar skin proximal to that joint. The skin of the radial palm is supplied by the palmar cutaneous branch of the median nerve proximal to the carpal tunnel. The autonomous zone of the median nerve is the index finger tip (Figure 3-32). The thumb can display some sensory overlap from the dorsoradial sensory nerve and even terminal branches of the lateral antebrachial cutaneous nerve. There can be some variability in the innervation of the ring and long finger between the median and ulnar nerves.

The ulnar nerve supplies the entire small finger and the ulnar half of the ring finger. This includes the palmar and dorsal skin from the tips to the level of the proximal interphalangeal joints and the palmar skin proximal to those joints. The skin along the dorsoulnar portion of the hand, and up to the level of the proximal interphalangeal joints of the ring and small fingers, is supplied by the dorsoulnar sensory nerve branch proximal to the wrist. The autonomous zone of the ulnar nerve is the small fingertip.

The dorsoradial sensory nerve branch of the radial nerve supplies the dorsoradial surface of the hand to the level of the proximal interphalangeal joints of the index and middle fingers and the thumb. The autonomous zone is the dorsal webspace between the thumb and index digits.

The majority of sensory testing is based on subjective responses. For this reason, it is important that the patient understand what is being tested and how it will be performed.

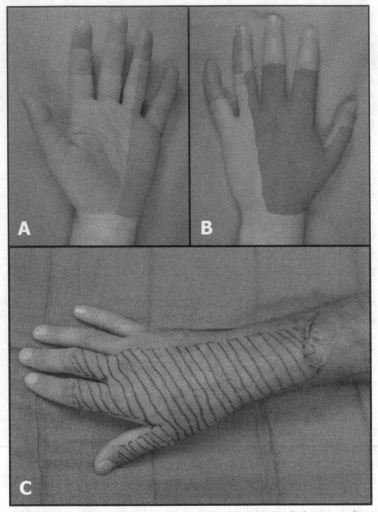

Figure 3-32. (A) Innervation of the hand palmarly divided into median and ulnar nerve distribution. (B) Innervation of the hand dorsally with dorsal hand innervated by dorsoradial sensory nerve and dorsoulnar sensory nerve. (C) Patient with dorsoradial sensory nerve laceration illustrating area affected.

Repeated testing of the same area helps to determine consistency and accuracy.

As the nerves and their mechanoreceptors possess unique physical properties, the tests assessing their function are also

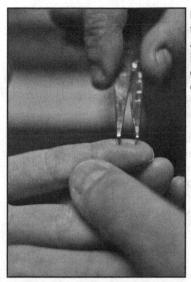

Figure 3-33. Instruments used to test two-point discrimination can be as simple as a paper clip unbent into 2 separate points. The minimal distance at which the patient can distinguish two points is noted.

unique. Touch sensation is evaluated by testing innervation density and threshold testing. Innervation density varies with the area of the body being tested. Static two-point discrimination is a good test for innervation density and is served by slowly adapting nerve fibers and their Merkel complex. There are various instruments that have been devised to help measure two-point discrimination (Figure 3-33). These are used to ascertain at what distance the patient can resolve the difference between those two separate points. The testing is performed along the palmar-lateral aspect of the pump of the fingertip so as to examine the radial and ulnar digital nerves separately. Exert enough pressure with the points of the device to blanch the skin. There can be some individual variability, with most individuals having the ability to distinguish two points at less than 6 mm. Moving two-point discrimination is performed by moving the instrument along the border of the digit. This is a good assessment of quickly adapting nerve fibers and their Meissner's corpuscles. Both of these tests can be used to assess nerve function and document recovery following nerve injury.

Threshold testing is performed with vibratory testing and Semmes-Weinstein monofilaments. Monofilament testing is performed by exerting a set amount of pressure on the pulp

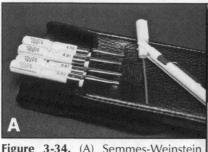
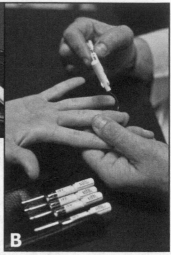

Figure 3-34. (A) Semmes-Weinstein monofilaments are plastic filaments of varying thickness. (B) Monofilaments are applied to the fingertip until they bend, and the patient is asked if he or she can feel the pressure.

of the fingertip using monofilaments of varying thickness. This is perceived by the slowly adapting nerve fibers and their Merkel complex bodies (Figure 3-34). Vibratory testing is performed at both low (30 Hz) and high (256 Hz) frequencies. A tuning fork is applied to the fingertip after it is activated, and the patient is asked to respond when the stimulus ceases. This information is provided by quick adapting nerve fibers and their Meissner's and Pacinian corpuscles.

Threshold testing is best for assessing subtle nerve changes or abnormalities that occur over time. Innervation density testing is best for gross testing after acute injury or to measure recovery over time.

If the patient cannot cooperate with the sensory examination (children, unconscious patient), the "pruning reflex" can be used. By immersing the hand and digits in water, the portions of skin that are normally innervated will elicit a normal pruning reflex while those that are not will stay smooth.

REFERENCES

1.   Malik AK, Morris T, Chou D, Sorene E, Taylor E. Clinical testing of ulnar collateral ligament injuries of the thumb. *J Hand Surg Eur.* 2009;34(3):363-366.

2.   Medical Research Council. Aids to the examination of peripheral nervous system. London, UK: Her Majesty's Stationary Office; 1976.
3.   Mathiowetz V, Kashman N, Volland G, Weber K, Dowe M, Rogers S. Grip-and-pinch strength: normative data for adults. *Arch Phys Med Rehabil.* 1985;66(2):69-74.
4.   Tredgett MW, Pimble LJ, Davis TRC. The detection of feigned hand weakness using the five position grip strength test. *J Hand Surg.* 1999;24B:426-428.
5.   Hildreth DH, Breidenbach WC, Lister GD, et al. Detection of submaximal effort by use of the rapid exchange grip. *J Hand Surg.* 1989;14A:742-745.
6.   Joughlin K, Gulati P, Mackinnon SE, et al. An evaluation of rapid exchange and simultaneous grip tests. *J Hand Surg.* 1993;18A:245-252.
7.   Tredgett MW, Davis TRC. Rapid repeat testing of grip strength for detection of faked hand weakness. *J Hand Surg.* 2000;25B:372-375.

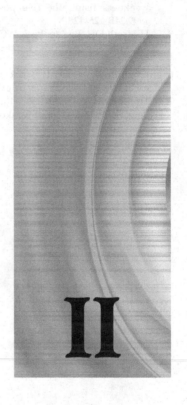

II

General Imaging

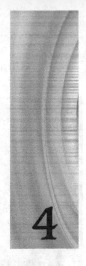

GENERAL IMAGING OF THE ELBOW

Hiu Yan Miranda Lai, MBChB, FRCR, MMed;
Amy F. Austin, MD; Kristen E. McClure, MD; and
William B. Morrison, MD

INTRODUCTION

Conventional radiography is typically the first imaging study in evaluating patients with elbow pain. In the appropriate clinical setting, ultrasound, computed tomography (CT), magnetic resonance imaging (MRI), and arthrography are invaluable in the evaluation of the elbow. This chapter will outline advantages of imaging techniques for different clinical conditions.

Culp RW, Jacoby SM. *Musculoskeletal Examination of the Elbow, Wrist, and Hand: Making the Complex Simple* (pp. 73-94). © 2012 Taylor & Francis Group.

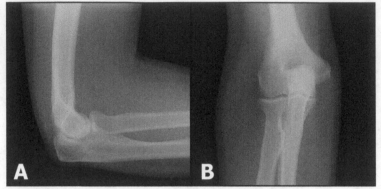

Figure 4-1. (A) Normal lateral and (B) frontal radiographs.

IMAGING MODALITIES

Radiography

Most evaluations of the elbow begin with radiographs because of their rapid acquisition, wide availability, and relatively low cost. Standard radiographic examination of the elbow includes an anteroposterior view, a true lateral view (Figure 4-1), and oblique views. The "radial head" view is obtained when there is clinical suspicion of radial head/neck fracture or early arthropathy that could be occult on standard views.

Assessment of the fat planes in true lateral view is essential. Elevation of the anterior and posterior fat pads is indicative of joint effusion; in the setting of acute trauma, underlying fracture is likely (Figure 4-2).[1] In setting of arthritis, displacement of the fat pads may indicate synovitis.

Other than the osseous details and fat planes, radiographs should also be evaluated for soft-tissue calcifications, which may indicate the presence of an intra-articular body (Figure 4-3), calcific tendonitis, calcific bursitis, or myositis ossificans.

Computed Tomography

With the advent of multi-detector computed tomography (MDCT), volumetric imaging data can be quickly acquired.

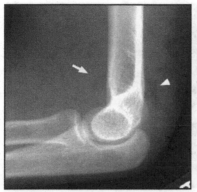

Figure 4-2. Elbow joint effusion. Lateral radiograph demonstrating elevation of the anterior fat pad (arrow) and posterior fat pad (arrowhead) related to elbow joint effusion.

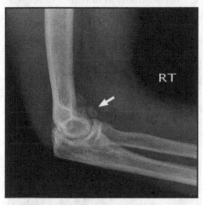

Figure 4-3. Intra-articular bodies. Lateral radiograph demonstrating large ossified intra-articular bodies (arrow).

Multiplanar reformats, three-dimensional reconstructions (Figure 4-4), and surface rendering are now possible and enable better delineation of the complex osseous anatomy and alignment of the elbow.

CT examination can detect the full extent of osseous injury that could be radiographically occult or obscured. The degree of angulation or amount of articular surface step-off can be accurately evaluated as well. Even if the injured elbow is stabilized within a cast in a flexed position, curved reformat technique enables "virtual" straightening of the arm for better assessment.

In addition, CT is highly sensitive in detecting calcium. Thus, it is very helpful in the detection of intra-articular bodies, characterization of bone tumors (for matrix, margins, and

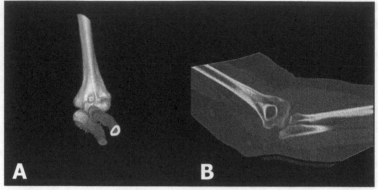

Figure 4-4. (A) Three-dimensional CT reconstruction and (B) curved CT multiplanar reformat demonstrating elbow dislocation.

Figure 4-5. Lateral fluoroscopic spot image during elbow arthrography demonstrating intra-articular contrast coursing around the capitellum.

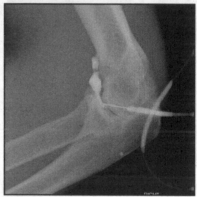

cortical breakthrough), and description of the character and extent of soft-tissue calcifications or ossifications.

Arthrography

Conventional elbow arthrography is now rarely used in isolation, but is typically combined with magnetic resonance imaging ([MRI] or direct MR arthrography) or CT (CT arthrography). Elbow arthrography combined with either of these modalities is helpful in diagnosing capsular and ligament tears, osteochondral lesions, and loose bodies.

With the use of a fluoroscopy table or C-arm, the joint can be entered laterally via the radiocapitellar joint (Figure 4-5). When a question of radial collateral ligament injury is present,

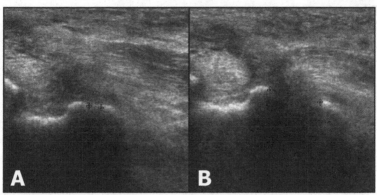

Figure 4-6. Coronal ultrasound of the medial elbow demonstrating ulnar collateral ligament laxity (A) before and (B) after valgus stress is applied to the elbow joint. The calipers measure the joint space between the ulna and trochlea.

posterolateral approach between the olecranon and the humerus could be employed. A 1.5 inch, 20- or 22-gauge needle is used to access the joint, and 7 mL to 10 mL of injectate (dilute gadolinium for MRI and iodinated contrast for CT) is then instilled, followed by imaging.

Ultrasound

Ultrasound (US) of the elbow is useful in evaluating a variety of conditions. In addition to the general assessment of joint effusions, loose bodies and regional bursae, the common extensor and flexor tendon, the medial collateral ligament, the distal biceps and triceps tendon, and the nerves can be evaluated in detail, facilitated by high-resolution linear array US probes. US scan of the elbow, as with other musculoskeletal US examinations, is best used as a focused examination about a specific anatomic structure based on clinical findings.

A particular strength of US is the ability to evaluate the dynamic status of anatomic structures in real time, when external stress is applied (Figure 4-6). This can be used for evaluation of subluxation of a tendon or a nerve or to evaluate functionality of a tendon or ligament (eg, MCL insufficiency in a throwing athlete).

Table 4-1

APPLICATIONS OF ELBOW ULTRASOUND

- Distal biceps and triceps tendon injuries assessment

- Evaluation of common flexor/extensor tendon injury

- Dynamic evaluation of medial collateral ligament insufficiency/tear

- Evaluation of ulnar nerve and cubital tunnel in ulnar neuropathy; detection of nerve subluxation on flexion and extension

- Evaluation of the radial and median neurovascular bundles for impingement and other conditions

- Articular assessment including joint effusions, intra-articular loose bodies and synovitis

- Ultrasound-guided joint aspiration or injection, and synovial and soft tissue biopsies

The major disadvantage of US examination is reliance on operator skill and expertise. Second, US provides excellent spatial resolution but is inferior in contrast resolution and global joint evaluation when compared with MRI. Moreover, due to the limitation of US penetration, deeper structures and osseous abnormalities are less accurately defined compared with CT and MRI.

Applications of US at the elbow are depicted in Table 4-1.

Magnetic Resonance Imaging

MRI plays a key role in directed or global assessment of the elbow. It displays normal anatomy in multiple planes. It is excellent in demonstrating bone, tendon, ligament, articular cartilage, and muscle anatomy and pathology.

Dedicated circumferential elbow surface coils, small field of view (12 to 14 cm), and high field-strength magnets provide optimal image quality. Image planes and field of view for the elbow vary with study indication and include axial, sagittal, and coronal planes; oblique and reformatted thin-section gradient-echo images are optional. The axial image plane is useful to assess neurovascular, tendon, and muscle anatomy. The sagittal plane is useful in evaluation of the anterior and posterior compartment structures and to define the extent of a lesion identified on axial images. The coronal plane is useful for evaluating articular surfaces, common extensor and flexor tendons, and collateral ligaments.

MRI accurately depicts osseous abnormalities, such as radiographically occult fractures and osteochondral injuries of the capitellum or the radial head. The osseous structures should be evaluated in every imaging plane, for bone marrow edema/replacement and cortical disruption. T1-weighted imaging is useful for depicting anatomy and marrow abnormalities. Fluid-sensitive imaging sequences (T2-weighted or sagittal fluid-sensitive sequence [STIR]) are best at visualizing fluid and edema in pathological conditions. Suspected tumors and infection are best evaluated by MRI.

Nuclear Medicine

Bone scintigraphy is a sensitive and efficient method of measuring metabolic activity of the entire skeleton. The mechanism of uptake is directly related to blood flow and degree of osteoblastic activity. It is extremely sensitive for detecting occult fractures, bone neoplasms, and infection. Nonetheless, it is relatively nonspecific and low resolution and is therefore rarely used for diagnosing disorders of the elbow.

PATHOLOGY

Acute Trauma

Radiography is the first imaging study performed in the setting of acute trauma. Most fractures and dislocations can be clearly depicted on standard conventional radiographs, although some fractures can be radiographically occult or obscured given the complex anatomy of the elbow. Additional oblique/radial head views may be performed to uncover the fracture lines or cortical deformity.

The "elevated fat pad sign" should always be looked for in the lateral view to assess the presence of a joint effusion. The

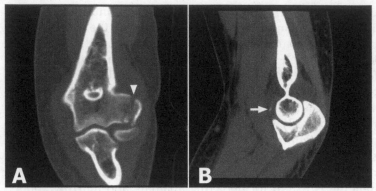

Figure 4-7. Coronal and sagittal CT reformatted images demonstrating (A) fracture of the capitellum with intra-articular extension and (B) an intra-articular osteochondral fragment.

absence of a joint effusion in an otherwise normal examination virtually eliminates the possibility of an occult fracture, whereas an effusion in the setting of trauma indicates a fracture until proven otherwise.[1]

CT examination can be very helpful in describing the full extent of osseous injury (Figure 4-7) and can detect fractures that are occult or obscured radiographically. The articular surfaces are better delineated on CT images. In cases of comminuted fractures and avulsion fractures, small osseous fragments are more readily demonstrated on CT.

MRI may be indicated in the setting of fracture or suspected dislocation for evaluation of soft-tissue involvement. MRI is capable of depicting both soft-tissue and osseous injuries as well as osteochondral abnormalities. Determining the presence of nerve and blood vessel involvement is particularly crucial in surgical planning. In pediatric patients, MRI can be used to evaluate disruption of cartilaginous epiphyseal and apophyseal structures that are radiolucent.

Overuse Injuries

Medial and Lateral Epicondylitis

Injuries of the common flexor and extensor tendons are generally referred to as medial and lateral epicondylitis, respectively. These injuries typically result from overuse of the particular muscle groups in occupational or sports-related

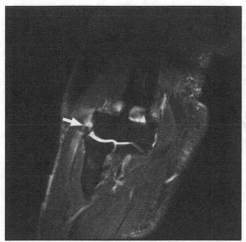

Figure 4-8. Lateral epicondylitis. Coronal fluid-sensitive image (T2 with fat suppression) demonstrating thickening and abnormal signal of the common extensor origin with partial-thickness tearing (arrow).

activities. They are usually diagnosed based on medical history and physical examination.

Radiographs are often performed to evaluate for associated pathology such as ossification at the tendon origin (enthesis) or underlying osteoarthropathy.

US may be used to visualize the degenerated tendons for tear[2]; the tendon will appear thickened with loss of normal fibrillar pattern and a heterogeneous appearance, possibly with shadowing calcifications. Doppler examination can be used to show areas of hyperemia. A partial-thickness tear appears as a focal nonshadowing anechoic area within the substance of the tendon, whereas a full-thickness tear demonstrates discontinuity and retraction of the tendon.

Although in most cases an MRI scan is not necessary, it should be considered in individuals with atypical symptoms or in patients who do not adequately respond to conservative measures. MRI is sensitive and specific in the evaluation of both medial and lateral epicondylitis (Figure 4-8) as well as underlying ligament tear.[3,4] Tendinosis is seen on MRI as diffuse increase in signal on T1- and T2-weighted images; tears are seen as focal fluid signal within the tendon. MRI also allows accurate assessment of the muscles, ulnar nerve, and collateral ligaments for concomitant pathology.

Figure 4-9. Partial-thickness tear of the ulnar collateral ligament. Coronal fluid-sensitive image (T2 with fat suppression) demonstrating abnormal signal about the distal aspect of the ulnar collateral ligament (UCL) with partial-thickness tearing (arrow).

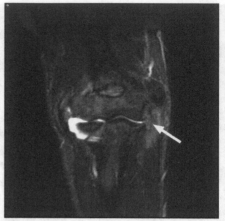

Ulnar Collateral Ligament Injury

Ulnar collateral ligament (UCL) injuries are most likely to occur in the setting of acute or chronic valgus stress, the latter being especially prevalent in overhead throwing athletes.

Radiography can occasionally show secondary findings that are suggestive of UCL injury, such as an avulsion fragment or ossification of the ligament. Additional manual or instrumented valgus stress radiography can be used to document medial joint opening and ligamentous laxity.

US is useful to evaluate the status of the UCL. It is capable of differentiating between a partial-thickness tear and a full-thickness tear and is also capable of demonstrating chronic changes related to repetitive trauma. One of the main benefits of US examination is the use of dynamic imaging, which can demonstrate laxity of the UCL and widening of the elbow during applied valgus stress.

MRI or MR arthrography can be used to demonstrate UCL injuries.[3,5] Coronal fluid-sensitive images are the best in demonstrating pathology (Figure 4-9); fluid located between the deep fibers of the UCL and its attachment to the adjacent bone is specific for a partial-thickness tear at the distal attachment site. A full-thickness tear is usually demonstrated as discontinuity of the fibers at midsubstance with joint fluid extravasation. MR arthrography allows for improved sensitivity by distending the joint recesses and is especially useful for detecting subtle undersurface tears.

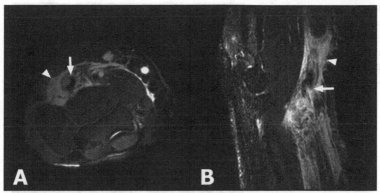

Figure 4-10. Distal biceps tendon rupture. (A) Axial and (B) sagittal fluid-sensitive sequences (T2 with fat suppression and STIR, respectively) demonstrate distal biceps tendon rupture with tendon retraction (arrow) and surrounding edema (arrowhead).

Muscle Injuries

Distal Biceps Brachii Tendon Injury

Radiography plays little or no role in the evaluation of the suspected distal biceps tendon tear, as there is usually no associated osseous avulsion fragment.

Distal biceps tendon injury can be detected on sonography. The end of the ruptured distal biceps tendon is surrounded by fluid and hemorrhage. A partial-thickness tear can be more difficult to identify but appears as a hypoechoic defect in an otherwise intact tendon. Occasionally, a complete tear shows no retraction if the overlying lacertus fibrosus remains intact. Differentiation of this condition versus a partial tear can be made by observing the tendon during active pronation and supination; if the tendon is completely torn, it will not slide back and forth.

MRI can accurately distinguish complete versus incomplete tear of the biceps tendon as well as the quality of the residual fibers and the extent of tendon retraction. Evaluation of the distal biceps tendon is best performed on sagittal and axial T2-weighted images with fat suppression (Figure 4-10).[6] The examination request should indicate imaging at the level of the elbow (so that the distal attachment site of the biceps tendon

Figure 4-11. Distal triceps avulsion. STIR demonstrating triceps tendon retraction (arrow) with an avulsed osseous fragment (arrowhead).

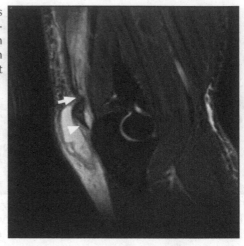

on the radial tuberosity is included), instead of imaging the upper arm where the resultant muscle bulge occurs.

Triceps Tendon Injury

Acute triceps tendon rupture is rare, usually occurring during a fall on an outstretched hand with excessive stress placed on the contracted muscle. In many cases, avulsion fracture of the olecranon occurs. Radiographs can help identify the avulsed bone fragments.

Clinically, it may be difficult to diagnose a partial tendon tear when there is overlying traumatic olecranon bursitis. Sonography may demonstrate discontinuity of the triceps tendon fibers in cases of tendon injury on longitudinal scan of the posterior aspect of the elbow. With complete rupture of the triceps tendon, absence of the tendon is noted with a fluid-filled gap. Avulsed olecranon process fragments may be seen as an echogenic focus with posterior shadowing.

MRI shows the triceps tendon best on T2-weighted sagittal images, whereas T2-weighted axial images are complementary.[6] On MRI, tendonitis appears as thickening and increased signal within the distal triceps tendon. Partial-thickness tear demonstrates fluid signal within the expected location of the tendon, and the tendon may be attenuated. A complete tear shows a fluid gap; MRI can determine the extent of retraction and the quality of the torn tendon end (Figure 4-11).

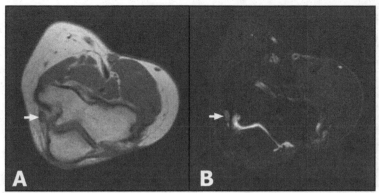

Figure 4-12. Ulnar neuropathy. (A) Axial T1 and (B) T2 fat-suppressed sequences demonstrate enlargement and abnormal signal of the ulnar nerve (arrow).

Ulnar Neuropathy

Cubital Tunnel Syndrome

The elbow is the second most common site of nerve entrapment in the upper extremity; the first being the wrist (carpal tunnel syndrome). Although the diagnosis of ulnar nerve entrapment at the elbow relies primarily on clinical and electrodiagnostic findings, in certain cases, MRI may establish the cause of the condition and provide crucial information for conservative management or surgical planning.

MRI is commonly used in the evaluation of peripheral nerve entrapment disorders to document signal and configuration changes in nerves and to evaluate for the presence of mass effect and distal muscle atrophy.[7] Fluid-sensitive fat-suppressed sequences best demonstrate abnormal edema signal within the nerve. Enlargement of the ulnar nerve proximal to the cubital tunnel with edema is indicative of cubital tunnel impingement (Figure 4-12). Although frank nerve compression may not be visible on MRI sequences acquired in extension, the source of nerve compression should be sought. Accessory anconeus epitrochlearis muscle, ganglion cyst, medial epicondylar spurs, joint synovitis, and post-traumatic soft-tissue infiltration are common sources of nerve compression in the cubital tunnel, and they are readily demonstrated on MRI.

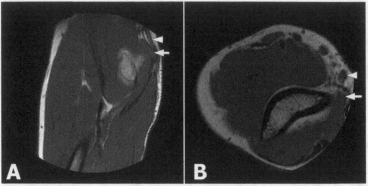

Figure 4-13. Snapping triceps and subluxing ulnar nerve. (A) Coronal and (B) axial T1 images demonstrate dislocation of the ulnar nerve (arrowhead) and subluxation of the medial bundle of the triceps (arrow).

Muscle denervation is seen as edema in the early stages with loss of muscle bulk, followed by fatty replacement.

Radiographs of the elbow may be helpful in documenting the source of ulnar nerve compression, such as osteophytes or other bone deformity. Ultrasound of the ulnar nerve focuses on the measurement of the short and long axes of the nerve at different levels with reference to the medial epicondyle. Enlargement of the nerve is suggestive of cubital tunnel syndrome.

Ulnar Nerve Dislocation and Snapping Triceps Syndrome

The ulnar nerve and medial head of the triceps muscle may dislocate over the medial epicondyle during elbow flexion[8] and produce a transient snapping sensation that is palpable at physical examination. Because ulnar nerve dislocation with and without accompanying snapping triceps syndrome may be clinically indistinguishable, imaging is often useful to assist in the diagnosis (Figure 4-13).

MRI sequences acquired at elbow extension may result in a false-negative assessment. Ultrasound is excellent for this purpose; observation of the cubital tunnel on active elbow flexion and extension can be used to document symptomatic nerve dislocation and correlate with the snapping sensation. If the source of snapping is unclear, the patient can be asked to

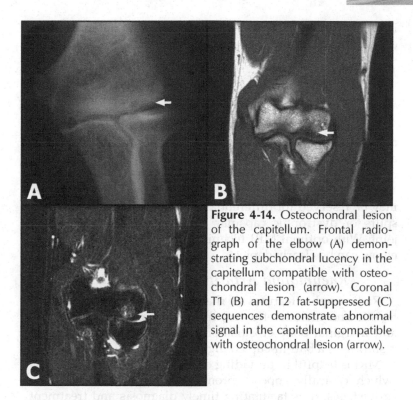

Figure 4-14. Osteochondral lesion of the capitellum. Frontal radiograph of the elbow (A) demonstrating subchondral lucency in the capitellum compatible with osteochondral lesion (arrow). Coronal T1 (B) and T2 fat-suppressed (C) sequences demonstrate abnormal signal in the capitellum compatible with osteochondral lesion (arrow).

reproduce the motion that generates the sensation with active sonographic visualization of the underlying anatomy.

Bone and Cartilage Pathology

Osteochondral Lesions

Osteochondral injury to the elbow usually occurs at the capitellum and is often related to chronic repetitive microtrauma caused by lateral impaction forces during valgus stress.

Radiographs may show irregularity or sclerosis of the articular surface; however, MRI is the imaging of choice for evaluation of osteochondral lesions (Figure 4-14).[3] It can accurately differentiate stable and unstable lesions; stable lesions have intact overlying cartilage whereas unstable lesions demonstrate a pattern of cartilage loss and fluid and cysts underlying the fragment. MR arthrography can increase the specificity in detecting unstable osteochondral lesions by demonstrating contrast surrounding the fragment.

Arthritis

Osteoarthropathy

Radiographic findings of osteoarthritis include joint space narrowing, subchondral sclerosis, subchondral cystic change, and osteophyte formation, usually at the anteromedial margin of the joint as well as the posterior margin at the olecranon.

MRI and CT scan are rarely required for diagnosis. They may be reserved for differentiating osseous loose bodies and spurs or dystrophic capsular ossification about the elbow joint. With optimal MRI technique, articular cartilage of the elbow can be clearly depicted.

Rheumatoid Arthritis

Radiographic features of rheumatoid arthritis are characteristic and include effusion, diffuse narrowing of the joint, and marginal bone erosions or even frank joint destruction resulting in a ball-in-cup configuration.

MRI is helpful in providing objective evidence of synovitis (which typically appears prominent and mass-like) in the early stages, thus facilitating timely diagnosis and treatment (Figure 4-15). Surrounding ligament and tendon tears can also be evaluated, potentially explaining new onset of pain. MRI also shows extra-articular soft-tissue consequences of the disease, including nodules on the extensor aspect of the elbow, swollen and entrapped nerves, and muscle changes resulting from nerve compression.[9] Ultrasound can also be used to evaluate synovitis and soft-tissue complications; additionally, Doppler evaluation can assess for underlying hyperemia due to inflammation.

Infection

Osteomyelitis

The olecranon is the most common site of bone infection in the elbow. Often, osteomyelitis is due to adjacent infectious bursitis or the consequence of local trauma in adult patients

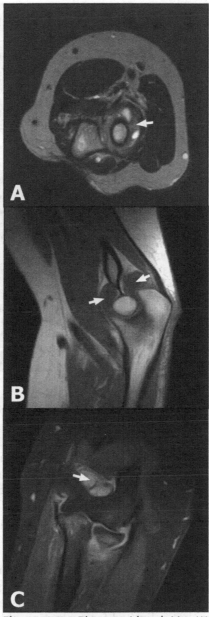

Figure 4-15. Rheumatoid arthritis. (A) Axial T2 (B) sagittal T1, and (C) coronal T2 fat-suppressed MR sequences demonstrating joint effusion with synovitis and pannus formation (arrows).

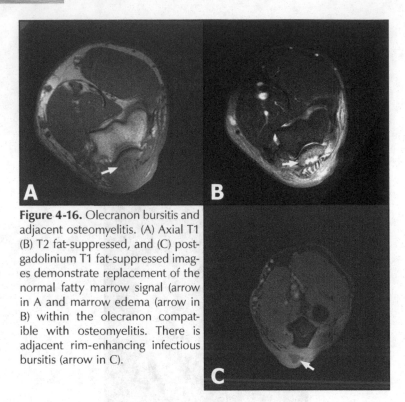

Figure 4-16. Olecranon bursitis and adjacent osteomyelitis. (A) Axial T1 (B) T2 fat-suppressed, and (C) post-gadolinium T1 fat-suppressed images demonstrate replacement of the normal fatty marrow signal (arrow in A and marrow edema (arrow in B) within the olecranon compatible with osteomyelitis. There is adjacent rim-enhancing infectious bursitis (arrow in C).

(Figure 4-16). In pediatric patients, hematogenous spread of infection is more common.

Acute osteomyelitis is first demonstrated radiographically by blurring or obliteration of soft-tissue fat planes, followed by intramedullary permeative destruction and indistinctness of the cortex. Although findings are characteristic, they often do not appear for 1 or 2 weeks after the onset of symptoms.[10]

MRI is much more sensitive to initial musculoskeletal changes and allows early diagnosis, and thus more effective use of antimicrobial therapy. It readily displays the presence of marrow edema and soft-tissue involvement. Contrast-enhanced imaging can be used to identify soft-tissue abscesses and sinus tracts. Ultrasound can be used to assess soft-tissue fluid collections but is limited for evaluation of bone involvement. A three-phase bone scan can be used for diagnosis of bone involvement but is limited in resolution and cannot be used to assess for soft-tissue abscess and other complications.

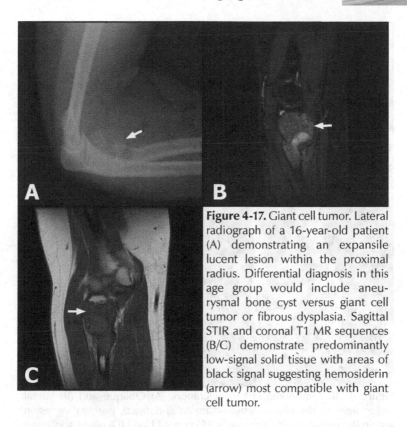

Figure 4-17. Giant cell tumor. Lateral radiograph of a 16-year-old patient (A) demonstrating an expansile lucent lesion within the proximal radius. Differential diagnosis in this age group would include aneurysmal bone cyst versus giant cell tumor or fibrous dysplasia. Sagittal STIR and coronal T1 MR sequences (B/C) demonstrate predominantly low-signal solid tissue with areas of black signal suggesting hemosiderin (arrow) most compatible with giant cell tumor.

Masses

Bone Tumor

Evaluation of suspected bone tumor in the elbow follows the general caveats for imaging of bone tumors elsewhere in the skeletal system. Radiographs are the first step of imaging and can distinguish aggressive and nonaggressive features of a bone lesion, allowing for generation of a limited differential diagnosis (Figure 4-17).[11]

CT is more sensitive than radiographs in detection of calcium and can be used to evaluate lesion margins, cortical interruption, bone destruction, and permeation as well as matrix mineralization, if not clearly demonstrated on radiographs.

MRI is accurate in determining local extent of a bone neoplasm (Figure 4-18). Multiplanar imaging facilitates local

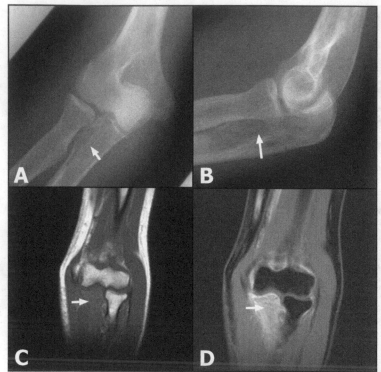

Figure 4-18. Lymphoma of the olecranon. (A) Oblique and (B) lateral radiographs of the elbow demonstrate an ill-defined, permeative lesion within the proximal ulna (arrows). (C) Coronal T1 and (D) post-gadolinium T1 fat-suppressed sequences demonstrate a mass replacing the normal marrow of the proximal ulna and olecranon with cortical breakthrough (arrows).

staging with improved preoperative and pretherapy assessment. Involvement of muscle compartments, joints, and neurovascular bundles can be readily evaluated. Moreover, MRI provides important information for determining site and route of biopsy, if warranted. Although MRI can be used to determine solid versus cystic nature of lesions, the imaging features are usually nonspecific in differentiating benign from malignant processes, and therefore MRI should not be ordered for this purpose.

Whole-body bone scintigraphy is efficient in screening the entire skeleton for multiplicity of lesions. However, bone scintigraphy is nonspecific in the diagnosis of bone tumors. Multifocality can be seen in some benign tumors (eg, fibrous dysplasia), and the amount of radiotracer uptake is not a reliable indicator of benignity or malignancy.

Recently, positron emission tomography (PET) has been found to be useful in following patients with bone and soft-tissue sarcomas after therapy. Fluorodeoxyglucose positron emission tomography (FDG-PET) has been shown to be able to distinguish recurrent tumor from post-therapeutic changes.

Soft-Tissue Masses

MRI is the image modality of choice for evaluation of a suspected soft-tissue mass because of its high spatial and contrast resolution in displaying soft-tissue anatomy. Multiple imaging planes can depict the compartmental location of the lesion and its relationship with adjacent fascial planes and neurovascular structures. Sometimes, specific diagnoses can be deduced based on location or tissue signal characteristics (eg, nerve sheath tumor, lipoma, ganglion cyst). When the diagnosis is in doubt and biopsy is warranted, MRI with contrast can depict areas of cystic or myxomatous change or necrosis, and thus guide the site of biopsy to solid regions.

In some cases, supplementary radiographs and CT may help in detecting and characterizing mineralization of soft-tissue lesions (eg, synovial sarcoma or myositis ossificans). Ultrasound has limited value in tissue characterization and global assessment of tissue involvement. However, either CT or US can be employed for image-guided biopsy if warranted.

REFERENCES

1. O'Dwyer H, O'Sullivan P, Fitzgerald D, et al. The fat pad sign following elbow trauma in adults: its usefulness and reliability in suspecting occult fracture. *J Comput Assist Tomogr.* 2004;28:562-565.
2. Connell D, Burke F, Coombes P, et al. Sonographic examination of lateral epicondylitis. *AJR Am J Roentgenol.* 2001;176:777-782.
3. Patten RM. Overuse syndrome and injuries involving the elbow: MR imaging findings. *AJR Am J Roentgenol.* 1995;164:1205-1211.
4. Thornton R, Riley GM, Steinbach LS. Magnetic resonance imaging of sports injuries of the elbow. *Top Magn Reson Imaging.* 2003;14:69-86.
5. Kaplan LJ, Potter HG. MR imaging of ligament injuries to the elbow. *Magn Reson Imaging Clin N Am.* 2004;12:221-232.

6. Chung CB, Chew FS, Steinbach L. MR imaging of tendon abnormalities of the elbow. *Magn Reson Imaging Clin N Am*. 2004;12:233-245.
7. Andreisek G, Crook DW, Burg D, et al. Peripheral neuropathies of the median, radial, and ulnar nerves: MR imaging features. *RadioGraphics*. 2006;26:1267-1287.
8. Jacobson JA, Jebson PJL, Jeffers AW, et al. Ulnar nerve dislocation and snapping triceps syndrome: Diagnosis with dynamic sonography— Report of three cases. *Radiology*. 2001;220:601-605.
9. Stoller DW. The elbow. In: Stoller DW (ed). *Magnetic Resonance Imaging in Orthopaedics and Sports Medicine*. 3rd ed. Philadelphia: Lippincott Williams & Wilkins; 2007:1613-1617.
10. Resnick D, Niwayama G. Anatomy of individual joints. In: *Diagnosis of Bone and Joint Disorders*. 4th ed. Philadelphia: WB Saunders; 1996.
11. Bancroft LW, Berquist TH, Peterson JJ, Kransdorf MJ. Imaging of elbow pathology. *Applied Radiology*. 2007;36:26-35.

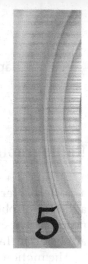

5

GENERAL IMAGING
OF THE WRIST

Frank E. Mullens, MD, MPH and William B. Morrison, MD

INTRODUCTION

Conventional radiography is almost always the first imaging study used in evaluating patients with wrist pathology. In the appropriate clinical setting, ultrasound, computed tomography (CT), magnetic resonance imaging (MRI), and arthrography are invaluable in the work-up as well. This chapter will outline advantages of imaging techniques for different clinical conditions.

Culp RW, Jacoby SM. *Musculoskeletal Examination of the Elbow, Wrist, and Hand: Making the Complex Simple* (pp. 95-120). © 2012 Taylor & Francis Group.

IMAGING MODALITIES

Radiography

Standard radiographic examination of the wrist includes a posteroanterior (PA) view and a lateral view,[1] usually with addition of oblique views and other supplementary views as needed.[2] These views may provide additional information and are listed in Table 5-1.

The motion of the wrist can also be observed actively under fluoroscopy (kinematic evaluation). The hand and forearm can also be placed under stress during fluoroscopic observation to visualize dynamic patterns of carpal instability that may not be apparent in the resting state. For example, axial load can be applied while the wrist is moved in flexion/extension (with lateral observation) or radial/ulnar deviation (observed in AP plane); or, if the patient reports symptoms of dynamic instability, the wrist can be observed fluoroscopically while the patient recreates the movement that incites the symptoms.[3]

Computed Tomography

With the advent of multi-detector computed tomography (MDCT), volumetric imaging data can be quickly acquired. Multiplanar reformats, three-dimensional reconstructions, and surface rendering are now possible and enable better delineation of the complex osseous anatomy and alignment of the wrist. Reconstructions can be performed in any plane without loss of information (ie, along the scaphoid to evaluate for healing fracture). CT examination can detect the full extent of osseous injury that could be radiographically occult or obscured. The degree of angulation or amount of articular surface step-off can be accurately evaluated as well. MDCT is particularly useful in acquiring images with minimization of metal artifact compared with older-generation CT scanners; this allows for accurate assessment of fixation for position, loosening, and other complications.[4]

In addition, CT is highly sensitive in detecting calcium. Thus, it is very helpful in detection of intra-articular bodies, subtle cortical erosions, characterization of bone tumors (for matrix, margins, and cortical breakthrough), and description of the character and extent of soft-tissue calcifications or ossifications.

Table 5-1

SUPPLEMENTARY WRIST RADIOGRAPHIC VIEWS AND USES

VIEW	TECHNIQUE	OPTIMALLY VISUALIZES
Supinated oblique view	Start with hand on its ulnar side; supinate 30 to 35 degrees	Pisiform and pisotriquetral joint
Pronated oblique view	Start with hand on its ulnar side; pronate 40 to 50 degrees	Scaphoid, triquetrum, scaphoid-trapezium-trapezoid (STT) and trapezium-trapezoid joints; body of hamate
Scaphoid view	Palmar surface of wrist placed on cassette Hand tilted in ulnar deviation x-ray beam tilted 20 degrees toward wrist	Scaphoid bone; view straightens scaphoid in frontal plane, allows better assessment of scaphoid fracture
Carpal tunnel view	Palmar surface of wrist placed on cassette Hand maximally dorsiflexed x-ray beam tilted 15 degrees toward palm	Pisiform, hamate hook; volar aspect of carpal bones
Radial/ulnar deviation views	AP views acquired with hand tilted in radial and ulnar direction	Carpal malalignment; views can accentuate joint widening or offset of carpal arcs in the setting of scapholunate or lunotriquetral ligament tear
Lateral flexion/extension views	Lateral views acquired with hand flexed and extended	Carpal malalignment; capitate should tilt with lunate; dissociation can indicate dynamic midcarpal instability

(continued)

Table 5-1 (continued)

Supplementary Wrist Radiographic Views and Uses

View	Technique	Optimally Visualizes
Closed fist view	Dorsal surface of wrist placed on cassette Fist clenched tightly Straight AP view acquired (can be in slight ulnar deviation)	Scapholunate interval; tension placed across carpus can widen joint in setting of interosseous ligament tear
Zero rotation view	Shoulder abducted 90 degrees Elbow flexed 90 degrees Forearm in neutral rotation Forearm flat on cassette x-ray beam centered at carpus; straight AP view	Ulnar variance; view straightens ulna and radius relative to each other, allows for assessment of positive or negative ulnar variance

Arthrography

Wrist arthrography is helpful in diagnosing tears of the triangular fibrocartilage complex (TFCC) as well as tears of the scapholunate (SL) and lunotriquetral (LT) ligament. Normally, these structures prevent fluid from passing into adjacent joint compartments; when they are torn or perforated, contrast will be seen to flow through. Injection should be observed actively so the location of the tear can be documented (ie, scapholunate versus lunotriquetral ligament tear). Injection is typically performed at the radiocarpal joint first (via the radioscaphoid joint from a dorsal approach) with injections into the midcarpal and distal radioulnar joint (DRUJ) if needed (after a delay to allow for resorption of radiocarpal contrast). However, it can be difficult to differentiate large tears from smaller perforations

Table 5-2

APPLICATIONS OF WRIST ULTRASOUND

- Carpal ganglion cyst
- Evaluation of common flexor/extensor tendon injury, tenosynovitis or tendinopathy
- Dynamic evaluation for tendon subluxation
- Evaluation of carpal tunnel syndrome
- Evaluation of the neurovascular bundles for impingement and other conditions
- Articular assessment including joint effusions, and synovitis

with plain arthrography; additionally, other important information—such as associated cartilage loss or other potential sources of pain—is lacking. Therefore, MRI has virtually supplanted plain arthrography. When performed, arthrography is typically combined with MRI (direct MR arthrography) or CT (CT arthrography); in this case, only a radiocarpal injection of contrast is performed.[5]

Ultrasound

Ultrasound of the wrist is useful in evaluating a variety of conditions.[6] In addition to the general assessment of joint effusion and synovitis, the extensor and flexor tendons (and the carpal tunnel) as well as the neurovascular structures including the median nerve are easily assessable. Ultrasound is an efficient way to perform a targeted exam, such as to confirm the presence of an occult ganglion cyst. The major disadvantage is reliance on operator skill and expertise. Also, ultrasound cannot evaluate osseous pathology and is limited to evaluation of deeper structures such as the TFCC and interosseous ligaments. For global joint evaluation or a less targeted exam (eg, "ulnar-sided pain"), MRI is optimal.

On the other hand, a particular strength of ultrasound is the ability to evaluate the dynamic status of anatomic structures in real time, with motion of the hand (ie, evaluation for subluxation of the extensor carpi ulnaris).

Applications of ultrasound at the wrist are depicted in Table 5-2.

Magnetic Resonance Imaging

MRI plays a key role in assessment of the wrist for global assessment as well as for targeted exams, such as for evaluation of ligament pathology or occult osseous injury.[7] Anatomy is depicted in multiple planes. MRI is excellent in demonstrating bone, tendon, ligament, articular cartilage, and muscle anatomy and pathology. However, scan quality can be variable based on scanner field strength and configuration. For high-quality imaging of any body part, a high field-strength scanner (ie, 1.0 Tesla or above) is recommended. However, for elbow, wrist, and hand/finger imaging, even high field scanners can provide low-quality imaging due to scanner configuration. An enclosed scanner requires the patient to place his or her arm either above his or her head in "Superman" position (an uncomfortable position in which to hold still for 30 to 40 minutes, resulting in motion artifact) or by his or her side against the inner wall of the gantry (necessitating use of a flexible receive-only coil yielding lower-quality images). For consistent image quality, high field open or wide bore scanners are available; there is even a 1.5 Tesla dedicated extremity MR scanner on the market.

Small field-of-view images (10 to 12 cm) are essential for evaluation of the wrist. The coronal plane is the "workhorse" plane, providing the best overall anatomic depiction of the osseous structures, effusions, carpal alignment, and ligamentous structures. Axial imaging plane is useful to assess carpal ganglion cysts, neurovascular, tendon, and muscle anatomy as well as dorsal and volar bands of the interosseous ligaments. The sagittal plane is useful as an additional plane to assess questioned abnormalities in the other planes in longitudinal orientation; it also provides limited assessment of radial-lunate-capitate alignment (although apparent alignment can be altered by hand positioning).

T1-weighted imaging is useful for depicting anatomy and marrow abnormalities. Fluid-sensitive imaging sequences (T2-weighted or STIR) are best at visualizing fluid and edema in pathological conditions. Suspected tumors and infection are best evaluated by MRI.

Nuclear Medicine

Bone scintigraphy is a sensitive and efficient method of measuring metabolic activity of the entire skeleton. The mechanism of uptake is directly related to blood flow and degree of osteoblastic activity. It is extremely sensitive for detecting occult fractures, bone neoplasms, and infection. Nonetheless, it is relatively nonspecific and low resolution, and is therefore rarely used for diagnosing disorders of the wrist.

Imaging Pitfalls

On any modality—but particularly x-ray, CT, and MRI—bony alignment can be altered by hand positioning. It should be understood that before diagnosing a subtle malalignment, the position in which images were acquired should be considered. For example, pronation and supination will alter relative length of the ulna and radius at the wrist. Flexion/extension and radial/ulnar deviation of the hand will appear to alter alignment as well. For example, radial deviation (fingers tilted toward the radial side) results in palmar flexion of the scaphoid and lunate, whereas ulnar deviation causes the scaphoid and lunate to dorsiflex. Volume averaging is another pitfall that occurs on CT and MRI. Each image represents a slice of certain thickness; if a structure is oblique to the imaging plane (ie, surfaces of the small bones of the carpus), signal will "average" with the adjacent structure (ie, joint fluid), and it will artificially appear abnormal or the margins will appear to "fade out."

PATHOLOGY

Acute Trauma

Similar to other joints, radiography should be the first imaging study performed in the setting of acute trauma. Most fractures and dislocations can be clearly depicted on standard conventional radiographs (Figures 5-1 and 5-2), although some fractures can be radiographically occult or obscured given the complex anatomy of the wrist. Additional views (see Table 5-1)

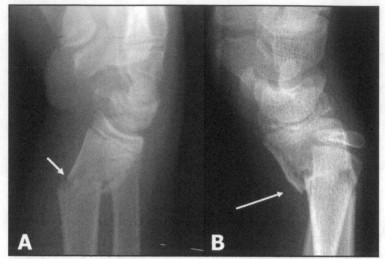

Figure 5-1. (A) Lateral radiographs of the wrist show dorsally angulated fracture of the distal radius (Colle's fracture). (B) Lateral radiograph of the wrist shows volarly angulated fracture of the distal radius (Smith's fracture).

Figure 5-2. Lateral radiograph of the wrist shows volar dislocation of the capitate with a normally positioned lunate consistent with perilunate dislocation.

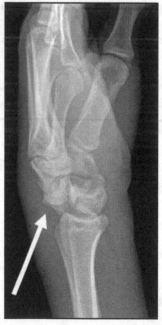

can be useful to optimally depict certain regions and uncover fracture lines or cortical deformity.[8]

Unlike the elbow, effusions at the wrist cannot be reliably diagnosed by radiographs. However, in the setting of trauma, any localized soft-tissue swelling should initiate a careful search for fracture or bony deformity in the region. If fracture is suspected but not seen on radiographs, a delay of 4 to 5 days with repeat radiographic examination can be useful; resorption of bone at the fracture site that occurs in the early phase of healing can make a fracture more obvious at this time. Because of the hyperemia and healing response that occurs with fractures, a triple bone scan can also be useful to detect fracture. Although highly sensitive, this test is not specific and will be positive with any process that induces bone turnover including inflammation, arthritis, and tumor; additionally, resolution is very low, and soft-tissue injury cannot be evaluated.

CT examination can be very helpful in describing the full extent of osseous injury prior to treatment and can be useful for detection of suspected fractures following negative radiographic evaluation. The complex articular surfaces of the carpal bones are better delineated on CT images. In cases of comminuted fractures and avulsion fractures, small osseous fragments are more readily demonstrated on CT.[4] Three-dimensional reconstructions facilitate surgical planning, especially with complex injury patterns (Figure 5-3).

Although other tests are also highly sensitive, MRI is the best single test for global evaluation of wrist injury. In the setting of negative radiographs but high suspicion, MRI easily detects fractures (Figure 5-4) and can also differentiate fractures from bone bruises (seen as bone marrow edema without a fracture line).[9] Unlike other modalities, soft-tissue injury (tendons, ligaments) can also be fully characterized.

Ligament Injury

Tears of the triangular fibrocartilage complex (TFCC) are generally not seen radiographically, although positive ulnar variance (a long ulna relative to the radius) and resultant ulnar abutment are highly suggestive of underlying ligament tear. Scapholunate and lunotriquetral ligament tear can be diagnosed on radiographs in the presence of associated joint widening or offset of the carpal arcs (Figure 5-5). Arthrography

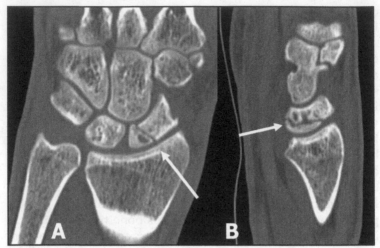

Figure 5-3. (A) Coronal and (B) Sagittal CT reconstructions of the wrist show carpal bone anatomy and demonstrate a proximal pole scaphoid fracture (arrows) with well corticated smooth edges characteristic of non-union with underlying subchondral cystic change spanning the fracture fragments.

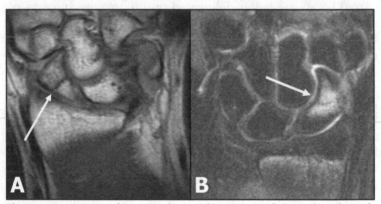

Figure 5-4. A) Coronal T1 MRI shows a hypointense fracture line through the midpole of the scaphoid (arrow). B) Coronal T2 fat-suppressed MRI (different patient) shows intense bone marrow edema (arrow) within the scaphoid characteristic of a fracture with a faint hypointense fracture line.

can be performed to diagnose communication between the radiocarpal and midcarpal compartments or the radiocarpal and DRUJ related to intervening ligament tear. However,

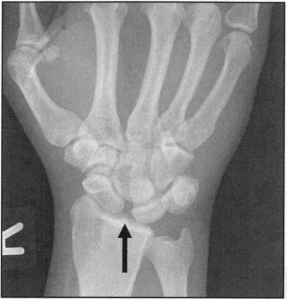

Figure 5-5. AP radiograph of the wrist shows marked widening of the scapholunate interval (arrow) consistent with scapholunate ligament tear.

overall, MRI is the best test for TFCC, scapholunate, and lunotriquetral ligament tear.[10] MR or CT arthrography (generally with contrast injected into the radiocarpal joint) provides excellent image quality (Figure 5-6) with the additional benefit of visualizing communication between compartments, but standard noncontrast high-resolution MRI performed on a high field system is usually all that is required (Figure 5-7).

Joint effusion in the DRUJ is highly suggestive of TFCC tear. Direct visualization on MRI is best performed in the coronal plane with fluid-sensitive sequences. On this sequence, TFCC tears are seen as areas of communication or discontinuity. Size of the tear as well as underlying central fibrocartilage thinning (suggesting a degenerative tear) should be reported (Figure 5-8). The periphery of the TFCC is composed of ligamentous attachments to the ulnar styloid and fovea; discontinuity or fluid extending across these bundles is diagnostic of peripheral tear (Figure 5-9). Fluid or synovitis in the ulnar

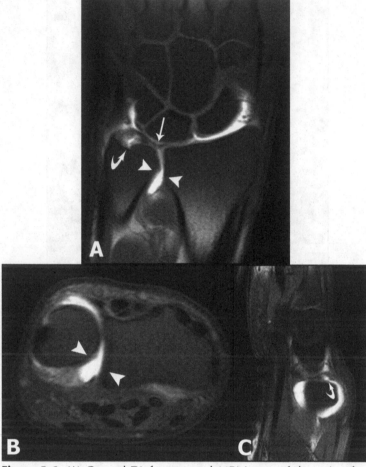

Figure 5-6. (A) Coronal T1 fat-saturated MRI image of the wrist after radioscaphoid joint intra-articular injection of dilute gadolinium-based contrast demonstrates contrast in the distal radioulnar joint (arrowhead), compatible with disruption of the TFCC, allowing contrast to enter the distal radioulnar joint (DRUJ). There is thinning and perforation of the central triangular fibrocartilage (solid arrow). There is also a tear involving the distal TFCC with tear of the ulnar foveal attachment (curved arrow). (B) Axial T1 fat-saturated MRI of the wrist shows a distal radioulnar joint effusion (arrowheads). (C) Sagittal T1 fat-saturated MRI of the wrist demonstrates a tear of the peripheral triangular fibrocartilage (TFC) at its peripheral attachment to the ulna.

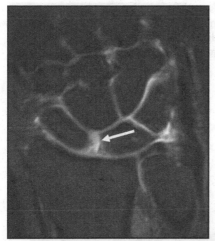

Figure 5-7. Coronal T2 fat-suppressed MRI shows complete tear of the scapholunate ligament (arrow).

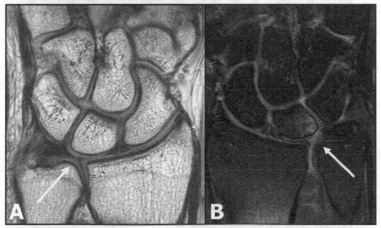

Figure 5-8. (A) Coronal T1 image shows slit-like perforation of the central TFCC (arrow). (B) Coronal T2 fat-suppressed image shows a large central degenerative tear of the TFCC (arrow) with associated osteoarthritic change.

recesses is also suggestive of tear as a secondary sign. For scapholunate and lunotriquetral ligament tear, coronal fluid-sensitive MRI sequences are also best; discontinuity is diagnostic of a tear but care should be taken to inspect the dorsal and volar bands to assess for a mechanically significant partial tear. Axial fluid-sensitive sequences are especially good for

Figure 5-9. Coronal T2 fat-suppressed MR image shows peripheral TFCC tear (thick arrow) with a distal radioulnar joint effusion (thin arrow).

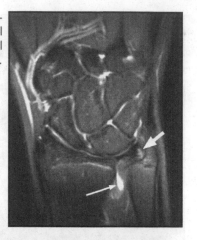

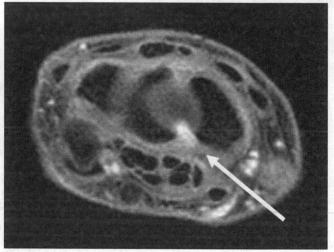

Figure 5-10. Axial T2 fat-suppressed MR image shows a partial tear of the volar bundle of the scapholunate ligament (arrow).

assessing the dorsal and volar bands (Figure 5-10). Smaller tears may not result in joint widening or offset.

Tendinopathy

Tendinopathy is best seen on ultrasound[11] or on MRI[12] with fluid-sensitive sequences in the axial plane. Tenosynovitis is seen as fluid in the sheath; associated synovial proliferation can be seen with an appearance of complex fluid or linear

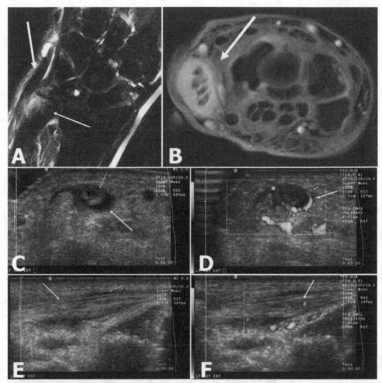

Figure 5-11. (A) Coronal T2 fat-suppressed MR demonstrates marked thickening of the extensor carpi ulnaris tendon with increased interstitial signal (arrow) with marked reactive bone marrow edema of the distal ulna. (B) Axial T2 fat-suppressed MR shows severe tenosynovitis of the first extensor compartment with tearing of the abductor pollicis longus and extensor pollicis brevis tendons. (C) Axial sonographic image of the wrist shows fusiform enlargement (thin arrow) and fluid surrounding (thick arrow) the first extensor compartment tendons characteristic of tendinosis with tenosynovitis. (D) Axial color Doppler sonographic images of the wrist at the same level show marked hyperemia (arrow). (E) Sagittal sonographic image of the wrist shows fusiform enlargement (thick arrow) and fluid surrounding (thin arrow) the first extensor compartment tendons characteristic of tendinosis with tenosynovitis. (F) Sagittal color Doppler sonographic image of the wrist at the same level shows marked hyperemia (arrow).

"synechiae" within the fluid. Tendinosis presents on imaging as thickening of the affected tendon with alteration of internal echogenicity (on ultrasound) or signal (on MRI) (Figure 5-11).

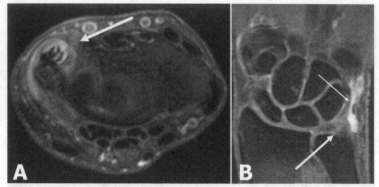

Figure 5-12. (A) Axial T2 fat-suppressed MR demonstrates marked thickening of the extensor carpi ulnaris tendon with split tear (arrow). (B) Coronal T2 fat-suppressed MR shows severe tenosynovitis of the extensor carpi ulnaris (thin arrow) with tearing of the peripheral TFCC (thick arrow).

Figure 5-13. Axial T2 MR image shows fluid signal surrounding the flexor tendons (arrow) consistent with severe tenosynovitis.

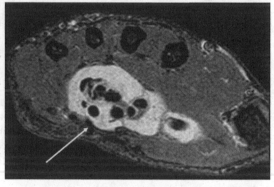

Traumatic tears may show underlying tendinopathy but more characteristically show focal discontinuity with normal adjacent tendon. The extensor carpi ulnaris tendon sheath is part of the TFCC, and tendinosis, tenosynovitis, or subluxation from the ulnar groove can be a secondary sign of peripheral TFCC tear (Figure 5-12).

Neuropathy

Neuropathy at the wrist can be related to the median nerve (at the carpal tunnel) or the ulnar nerve (at Guyon's canal). Carpal tunnel syndrome is typically related to tenosynovitis of the flexor compartment and is seen on ultrasound[13,14] or MRI[15] as fluid surrounding the tendons (Figure 5-13; flexor

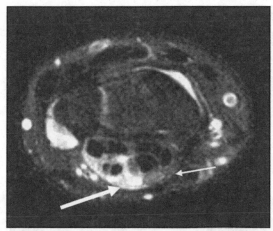

Figure 5-14. Axial T2 fat-suppressed MR image shows flexor tenosynovitis with bowing of the flexor retinaculum (thick arrow) with mild enlargement of the median nerve (thin arrow).

tenosynovitis); however, due to mass effect and constriction from the flexor retinaculum, the fluid can be squeezed from the central aspect of the tunnel and may only be observed proximally or distally. In more advanced cases, the median nerve will appear enlarged proximal to the carpal tunnel[16] with edema and prominent fascicles observed on transverse images (Figure 5-14). Similar findings of edema and enlargement can be seen at the ulnar nerve due to injury or impingement.[17] Neuromas can occasionally be observed with focal enlargement rather than the diffuse enlargement seen from impingement syndromes. Distal muscle atrophy can be seen in the distribution of the nerve with early edema and late fat replacement of the associated muscles.

Arthropathy

Inflammatory arthropathies are common at the wrist, in particular rheumatoid arthritis (RA). On radiographs, in the early stages, RA is seen as soft-tissue swelling, especially over the ulnar styloid, dorsum of the wrist, and the metacarpophalangeal (MCP) and proximal interphalangeal (PIP) joints. Rarefaction of bone is followed by erosive disease and diffuse cartilage loss with joint narrowing. Ultrasound can be useful for confirmation of synovitis and effusion but cannot evaluate the central aspects of the joints or underlying marrow. MRI can be used to acquire an overall picture of the extent

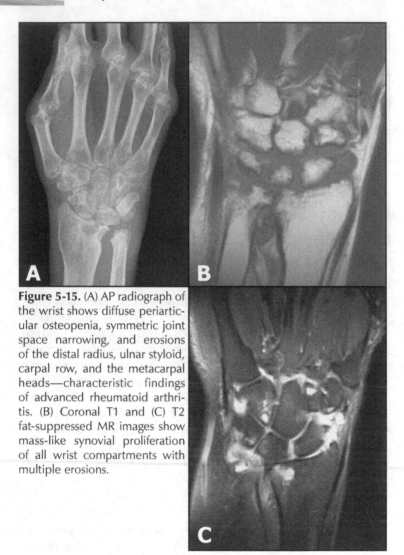

Figure 5-15. (A) AP radiograph of the wrist shows diffuse periarticular osteopenia, symmetric joint space narrowing, and erosions of the distal radius, ulnar styloid, carpal row, and the metacarpal heads—characteristic findings of advanced rheumatoid arthritis. (B) Coronal T1 and (C) T2 fat-suppressed MR images show mass-like synovial proliferation of all wrist compartments with multiple erosions.

of disease in the joints and other synovial compartments; RA typically presents on MRI as multifocal synovitis (ie, joints, tendon sheaths) with mass-like quality of synovial proliferation (Figure 5-15).[18]

Septic arthritis can affect the wrist with hematogenous spread but is more commonly due to penetrating trauma. Joint

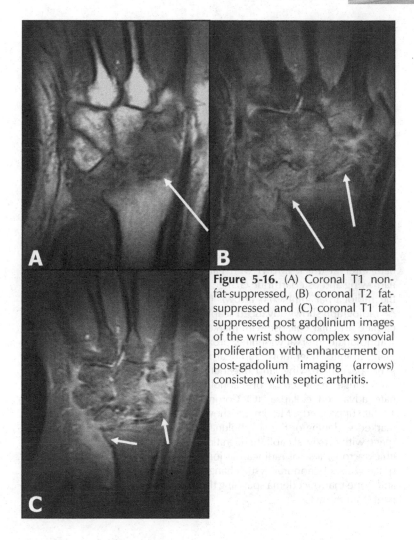

Figure 5-16. (A) Coronal T1 non-fat-suppressed, (B) coronal T2 fat-suppressed and (C) coronal T1 fat-suppressed post gadolinium images of the wrist show complex synovial proliferation with enhancement on post-gadolium imaging (arrows) consistent with septic arthritis.

effusion and synovial proliferation are characteristic, and the appearance is very similar on all imaging modalities to that of RA and other inflammatory arthropathies. MRI can be used to evaluate for bone marrow edema, which in the setting of septic arthritis suggests underlying osteomyelitis (Figure 5-16).

Degenerative arthritis at the wrist can be due to prior trauma (intra-articular fracture, interosseous ligament tear,

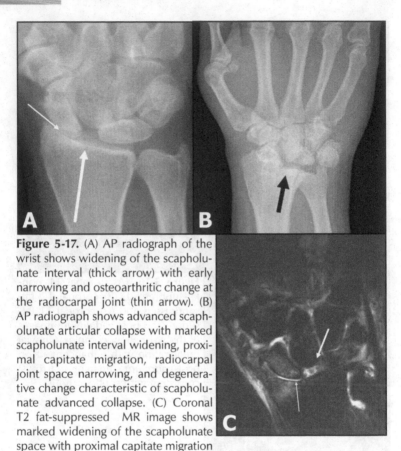

Figure 5-17. (A) AP radiograph of the wrist shows widening of the scapholunate interval (thick arrow) with early narrowing and osteoarthritic change at the radiocarpal joint (thin arrow). (B) AP radiograph shows advanced scapholunate articular collapse with marked scapholunate interval widening, proximal capitate migration, radiocarpal joint space narrowing, and degenerative change characteristic of scapholunate advanced collapse. (C) Coronal T2 fat-suppressed MR image shows marked widening of the scapholunate space with proximal capitate migration (thick arrow), loss of radiocarpal joint space with subchondral cystic change, and bone marrow edema spanning the joint (thin arrow).

etc) with malalignment or incongruity of articular surfaces. This is particularly common in the setting of scapholunate ligament tear with palmar flexion of the scaphoid and resultant scapholunate advanced collapse (SLAC) (Figure 5-17). Positive ulnar variance can also cause TFCC tear and osteoarthritis (OA) due to ulno-lunate abutment. Another common cause of OA is a type 2 lunate, with articulation on the proximal hamate, resulting in cartilage loss at the junction

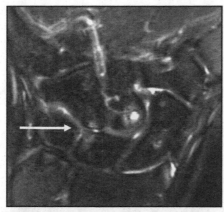

Figure 5-18. Coronal T2 fat-suppressed MR shows the hamate articulating with the lunate (Type II) with focal cartilage loss and subchondral cystic change across the articulation (arrow) consistent with secondary osteoarthritis.

(Figure 5-18). OA can also be due to cartilage loss related to prior inflammatory arthropathy. OA is seen radiographically as sclerosis, joint narrowing, and subchondral cystic change. On MRI, small to moderate effusions may be seen, with cartilage loss and subchondral edema representing various stages of cyst formation.

Joint Effusion/Recesses

MRI and ultrasound are the tests of choice for evaluation and characterization of ganglion cysts. Ganglia appear as lobulated fluid signal structures on MRI and rounded anechoic structures on ultrasound with increased through transmission. The neck should be sought to establish the origin. Although ganglia can occur off any synovial compartment, including tendon sheaths, they are most common at the dorsum of the wrist off the midcarpal region adjacent to the capitate/lunate joint and dorsal intercarpal ligament. Another common site is off the volar aspect of the radioscaphoid joint; these ganglia can dissect through the soft tissues to surround the radial artery (Figure 5-19).

Ganglia can also form adjacent to ligament tears; a cyst next to the TFCC or interosseous ligaments should raise suspicion for underlying ligament injury.

Knowledge of joint recesses and implications of effusions is also important. For example, the pisotriquetral recess is part

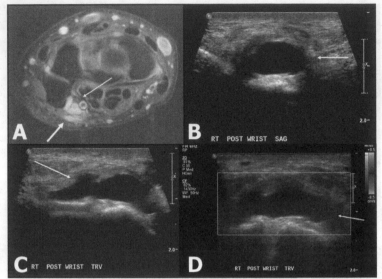

Figure 5-19. (A) Axial T2 fat-suppressed MR image demonstrates a hyperintense polylobulated fluid collection in Guyon's canal (thick arrow) consistent with a ganglion cyst with enlargement and increased signal within the adjacent ulnar nerve in a patient with ulnar neuritis (thin arrow). (B) Sagittal and (C) transverse sonographic images show a hypoechoic structure with increased through transmission (arrows) consistent with a ganglion cyst. (D) Findings are confirmed on sagittal Doppler image showing no internal vascularity in the cystic mass (arrow).

of the radiocarpal joint and can become distended, simulating a ganglion cyst on imaging exams. The ulnar recesses can normally contain small amounts of fluid, but the presence of synovitis suggests underlying TFCC tear. No fluid is normally present in the DRUJ, so any distension is suspicious for TFCC tear or other process (ie, arthropathy).

Tumor/Masses

The majority of perceived masses at the wrist actually represent benign processes such as ganglion cysts. Therefore, MRI without contrast (ie, a standard high-resolution wrist protocol) is indicated; contrast is generally not required. True masses may benefit from postcontrast imaging; solid tissue will enhance brightly, helping to differentiate cystic/necrotic

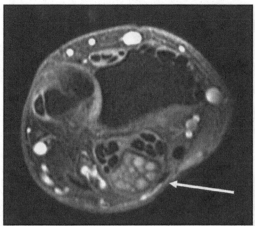

Figure 5-20. Axial T2 fat-suppressed MR shows marked enlargement of the median nerve with interspersed fat (arrow) consistent with a fibrolipomatous hamartoma.

tissue versus active tumor.[19] Ultrasound can also distinguish solid from cystic tissue, and Doppler evaluation can evaluate vascularity of the lesion as well as the relationship to adjacent blood vessels.[20] Occasionally, MRI can make a definitive diagnosis regarding origin of a solid mass (eg, monotonous fat signal in a lipoma or a lesion along a nerve representing a neuroma; Figure 5-20).

Avascular Necrosis/Kienböck's

The imaging appearance and progression of avascular necrosis is similar in all bones; in the early stages, radiographs and CT can appear normal. On MRI, the bone (or part of a bone, in the case of proximal pole scaphoid avascular necrosis [AVN] following fracture) appears diffusely edematous. In the lunate, generally, the whole bone is involved; "partial" AVN of the lunate is rare (proximal lunate edema is much more likely related to other causes such as ulnar impaction/abutment). In the early stages, some fat may be preserved on T1-weighted images, raising a differential diagnosis of hyperemic response to injury versus ischemia (especially in the scaphoid). If this is the case, a bolus of gadolinium contrast with rapid MR imaging can differentiate these phenomena.[21] In later stages, the bone becomes dense radiographically. If the extremity is immobilized, the adjacent bones can undergo resorption, making the avascular bone appear even more dense. However, a

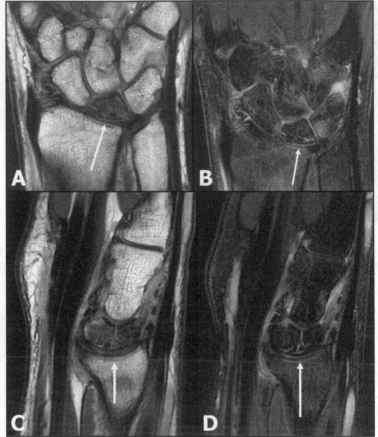

Figure 5-21. (A) Coronal T1 and (B) coronal T2 fat-suppressed and (C) sagittal T1 and (D) sagittal T2 fat-suppressed MR images show characteristic low signal marrow signal within the lunate characteristic of AVN (Kienböck's) with vertically oriented fracture line (arrow).

dense bone is not specific for AVN. On MRI, in this stage, the marrow fat often becomes replaced with calcium or fibrous tissue leading to a very dark appearance on all sequences, particularly gradient echo (GRE) images; however, edema signal may still be present. In later stages, avascular bone can undergo collapse or fragmentation with development of secondary osteoarthritis (Figure 5-21).

REFERENCES

1. Wheeless online (www.wheelessonline.com).
2. Russin LD, Bergman G, Miller L, et al. Should the routine wrist examination for trauma be a four-view study, including a semisupinated oblique view? *AJR Am J Roentgenol.* 2003;181:1235-1238.
3. Gilula LA, Destouet JM, Weeks PM, Young LV, Wray RC. Roentgenographic diagnosis of the painful wrist. *Clin Orthop Relat Res.* 1984;187:52-64.
4. Kaewlai R, Avery LL, Asrani AV, Abujudeh HH, Sacknoff R, Novelline R. Multidetector CT of carpal injuries: anatomy, fractures, and fracture-dislocations. *Radiographics.* 2008;28(6):1771-1784.
5. Moser T, Khoury V, Harris PG, Bureau NJ, Cardinal E, Dosch JC. MDCT arthrography or MR arthrography for imaging the wrist joint? *Semin Musculoskelet Radiol.* 2009;13(1):39-54.
6. Teefey SA, Middleton WD, Boyer MI. Sonography of the hand and wrist. *Semin Ultrasound CT MR.* 2000;21(3):192-204.
7. Zanetti M, Saupe N, Nagy L. Role of MR imaging in chronic wrist pain. *Eur Radiol.* 2007;17(4):927-938. Epub 2006 Aug 24.
8. Loredo RA, Sorge DG, Garcia G. Radiographic evaluation of the wrist: a vanishing art. *Semin Roentgenol.* 2005;40(3):248-289.
9. Brydie A, Raby N. Early MRI in the management of clinical scaphoid fracture. *Br J Radiol.* 2003;76(905):296-300.
10. Tananka T, Ogino S, Yoshioka H. Ligamentous injuries of the wrist. *Semin Musculoskelet Radiol.* 2008;12(4):359-377.
11. Jacob D, Cohen M, Bianchi S. Ultrasound imaging of non-traumatic lesions of the wrist and hand tendons. *Eur Radiol.* 2007;17(9):2237-2247.
12. Lisle DA, Shepherd GJ, Cowderoy GA, O'Connell PT. MR imaging of traumatic and overuse injuries of the wrist and hand in athletes. *Magn Reson Imaging Clin N Am.* 2009;17(4):639-654.
13. Buchberger W, Judmaier W, Birbamer G, Lener M, Schmidauer C. Carpal tunnel syndrome: diagnosis with high-resolution sonography. *AJR Am J Roentgenol.* 1992;159(4):793-798.
14. Sarría L, Cabada T, Cozcolluela R, Martínez-Berganza T, García S. Carpal tunnel syndrome: usefulness of sonography. *Eur Radiol.* 2000;10(12):1920-1925.
15. Mesgarzadeh M, Triolo J, Schneck CD. Carpal tunnel syndrome. MR imaging diagnosis. *Magn Reson Imaging Clin N Am.* 1995;3(2):249-264.
16. Yesildag A, Kutluhan S, Sengul N, et al. The role of ultrasonographic measurements of the median nerve in the diagnosis of carpal tunnel syndrome. *Clin Radiol.* 2004;59(10):910-915.
17. Zeiss J, Jakab E, Khimji T, Imbriglia J. The ulnar tunnel at the wrist (Guyon's canal): normal MR anatomy and variants. *AJR Am J Roentgenol.* 1992;158(5):1081-1085.
18. Boesen M, Ostergaard M, Cimmino MA, Kubassova O, Jensen KE, Bliddal H. MRI quantification of rheumatoid arthritis: current knowledge and future perspectives. *Eur J Radiol.* 2009;71(2):189-196. Epub 2009 May 27.

19. Ergun T, Lakadamyali H, Derincek A, Cagla Tarhan N, Ozturk A. Magnetic resonance imaging in the visualization of benign tumors and tumor-like lesions of hand and wrist. *Curr Probl Diagn Radiol.* 2010;39(1):1-16.
20. Bianchi S, Della Santa D, Glauser T, Beaulieu JY, van Aaken J. Sonography of masses of the wrist and hand. *AJR Am J Roentgenol.* 2008;191(6):1767-1775.
21. Schmitt R, Heinze A, Fellner F, Obletter N, Struhn R, Bautz W. Imaging and staging of avascular osteonecroses at the wrist and hand. *Eur J Radiol.* 1997;25(2):92-103.

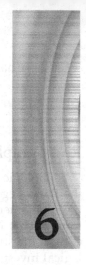

6

GENERAL IMAGING
OF THE HAND

John Shum Sing Fai, MBBS, FRCR and
William B. Morrison, MD

INTRODUCTION

The aim of this chapter is to assist the clinician in ordering the most appropriate radiological examination when imaging of the hand is deemed necessary. Advantages and disadvantages of different radiological modalities are first described. Further imaging techniques are also discussed in order to answer specific clinical questions.

Culp RW, Jacoby SM. *Musculoskeletal Examination
of the Elbow, Wrist, and Hand: Making the Complex
Simple* (pp. 121-137). © 2012 Taylor & Francis Group.

IMAGING MODALITIES

Radiography

Radiologic investigation of musculoskeletal pathology of the hand begins with radiographs. Radiographs provide initial assessment of trauma, arthritis, infection, and suspected tumor. This is a simple, low-cost tool that may answer the clinical question or, alternately, may help guide further radiological investigations. Standard views include anteroposterior (AP), lateral (with fingers splayed), and oblique if necessary. For rheumatoid arthritis, it may be useful to acquire a "ball-catcher's" or Norgaard view, which is an oblique frontal view of both hands.

Computed Tomography

Computed tomography (CT) allows excellent assessment of cortical bone. With the advance of multidetector CT (MDCT) and high-quality reformatting capability, accurate characterization of osseous pathology and different fracture patterns is facilitated. It is also a useful tool to evaluate for fracture union across metallic fixation, since metal artifact is minimized. However, CT is limited to evaluation of soft tissue pathology in the hand due to relatively poor contrast between soft tissue structures.

Ultrasound

Ultrasound (US) can be a powerful tool to assess superficial soft tissue structures or lesions of the hand (Table 6-1).[1] It is economic, quick, and allows real time performance of various stress maneuvers; for example, a trigger finger can be evaluated for catching of the tendon within a scarred portion of the sheath during active flexion and extension. US provides excellent depiction of foreign bodies that may not be visible on other imaging modalities. A high-frequency transducer must be used to acquire appropriate high-resolution images. Color-flow or power Doppler can provide demonstration of blood flow associated with neoplastic or inflammatory conditions (eg, to determine extent of synovitis in rheumatoid arthritis).

Table 6-1

APPLICATIONS OF ULTRASOUND FOR THE HAND

Tendon pathology

Soft tissue masses

Foreign bodies

Ligament Injury

Joint effusion/synovitis

In the context of masses, US is capable of defining solid and cystic areas (and for differentiating solid tumors versus ganglion cysts), defining the proximity to adjacent structures (eg, blood vessels), and determining whether a lesion is primarily vascular. Subsequent biopsies and aspirations can be performed using US guidance. However, evaluation of osseous and articular pathology on US is limited compared with CT and MR.

MAGNETIC RESONANCE IMAGING

Magnetic resonance imaging (MRI) allows noninvasive assessment of the anatomy and subtle pathological processes without the use of ionizing radiation. However, MRI of the hand can be technically challenging due to the small size of the structures being imaged and the fact that the surface coils used to acquire images of various body parts are not designed for hand imaging and are not optimized for this purpose. In order to acquire the best possible contrast and spatial resolution, small coils and high field strength (eg, 1.0 Tesla or greater) should be used (Figure 6-1). MRI is excellent for characterizing soft tissue masses for location and composition, and often a definitive diagnosis can be made. For example, a low-signal mass associated with a tendon sheath is typically a giant cell tumor of the tendon sheath. MRI is more sensitive than radiography in detecting early erosions of the hand and wrist in the

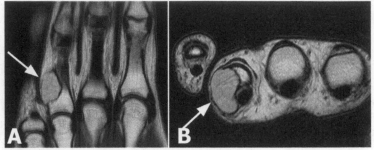

Figure 6-1. (A) High resolution coronal and (B) axial MR images of the finger using a dedicated high field-strength 1.5 Tesla extremity unit (GE Medical Systems). MR imaging of the hand and fingers can be challenging unless dedicated coils and high field (1.0 Tesla or higher) scanners are used. Imaging depicts a juxtacortical chondroma (arrow).

Table 6-2

APPLICATIONS OF HAND MAGNETIC RESONANCE IMAGING

Occult Fracture/bone bruise

Tendon Pathology

Ligament tear

Capsular injury

Arthritis

Ganglion cysts/soft tissue masses

Infection

setting of inflammatory arthropathy. MRI is also excellent for evaluation of other soft tissue pathology, such as tendinopathy and tenosynovitis, pulley injuries, capsular injuries, and ligament tears (Table 6-2).

MRI enables assessment of bone marrow and detection of radiographically occult injuries. However, MRI is less sensitive than radiographs for detection of small avulsion fractures.

Intravenous contrast can be used for evaluation of vascularity (of tumors or synovial processes), differentiating solid versus cystic lesions, evaluation of infection, and assessment of chronic injuries with scarring.

NUCLEAR MEDICINE

Nuclear medicine scans dedicated to the hand can be used to evaluate for numerous conditions such as arthralgias and reflex sympathetic dystrophy, as well as various types of radiographically occult osseous pathology. It may also be useful in determining multiplicity of lesions. A "three-phase" bone scan (with imaging of vascular, blood pool, and delayed uptake) can be useful for diagnosing infection. However, its use in the hand is limited by lack of specificity and spatial resolution.

CLINICAL INDICATIONS

Injury

Osseous Injury

For evaluation of suspected fracture, radiographs are essential (Figure 6-2); they provide a cheap, rapid overview of cortical discontinuity, avulsions, and alignment. If clinically necessary, MRI allows assessment of bone marrow and detection of radiographically occult injuries, as well as assessment of associated soft tissue injury. A combination of T1-weighted images and fluid-sensitive (STIR or fat-suppressed T2-weighted) images can differentiate bone bruise (ill-defined edema) from fracture (linear low T1 signal). However, small avulsion fractures may be difficult to detect.

CT is more often used in other regions where the osseous anatomy is more complex. It may be needed in special cases to evaluate complex fractures or those involving the articular surfaces in order to plan surgery. Reformatted 2-dimensional and 3-dimensional images can be acquired. Assessment of fracture healing and fixation loosening can be performed if not evident on radiographs (Figure 6-3).

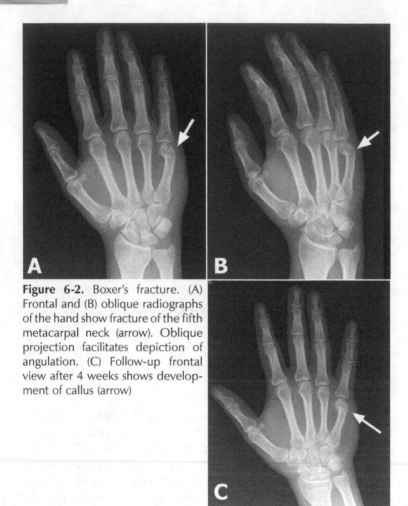

Figure 6-2. Boxer's fracture. (A) Frontal and (B) oblique radiographs of the hand show fracture of the fifth metacarpal neck (arrow). Oblique projection facilitates depiction of angulation. (C) Follow-up frontal view after 4 weeks shows development of callus (arrow)

Soft Tissue Injury

Tendon Injury

Acute tendon tear that is suspected clinically is best assessed using US or MRI (Figure 6-4).[1-4] These modalities can evaluate location and extent of tear (eg, percentage of the tendon torn in partial tears) and assess for associated soft tissue injuries. These modalities are also recommended for chronic tendon

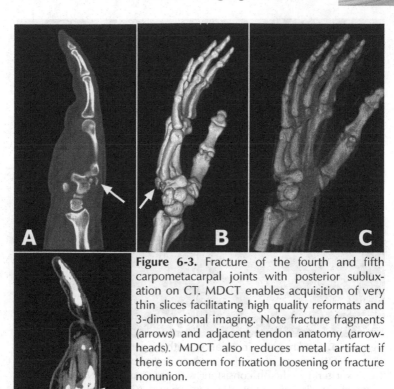

Figure 6-3. Fracture of the fourth and fifth carpometacarpal joints with posterior subluxation on CT. MDCT enables acquisition of very thin slices facilitating high quality reformats and 3-dimensional imaging. Note fracture fragments (arrows) and adjacent tendon anatomy (arrowheads). MDCT also reduces metal artifact if there is concern for fixation loosening or fracture nonunion.

pathology such as tendinosis (tendon thickening and intrinsic heterogeneity) and tenosynovitis (excess fluid or complex fluid in sheath). "Trigger finger" can be evaluated by dynamic US, with the location and cause of tendon catching observed in real time during motion.

Pulley Injuries

A series of fibrous bands or "pulleys" encircle the flexor tendons and help stabilize them during motion. Tears can be seen in chronic overuse or acute injury and are especially prevalent in rock climbers. US and MRI are effective means to demonstrate pulley injuries demonstrating disruption of the fibers and "bowstringing" of the tendon (Figure 6-5).[5,6]

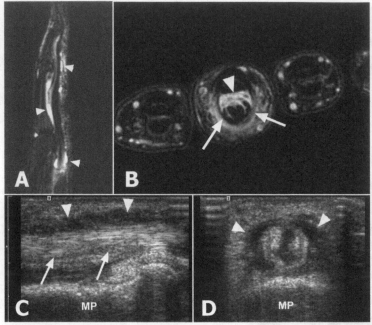

Figure 6-4. Tendinopathy in a patient with trigger finger. (A) Sagittal and (B) axial MR images of the finger show complex fluid (arrowheads) in the flexor tendon sheath consistent with tenosynovitis. Note intact but edematous pulley on the axial image (arrows). (C) Sagittal and (D) axial US images show anechoic fluid in the sheath (arrowheads). Note the thickened, irregular appearance of the degenerated tendon (arrow). US has the advantage of observing tendon catching in real time.

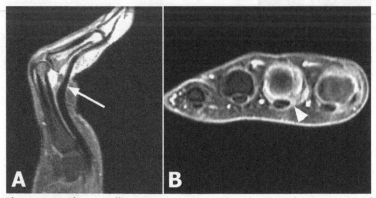

Figure 6-5. Flexor pulley injury. (A) Sagittal and (B) axial MR images of the finger show increased distance between the flexor tendon (arrow) and the proximal phalanx, the "bowstring deformity" related to an A2 pulley injury. Axial image shows disruption of the pulley (arrow).

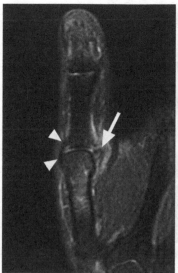

Figure 6-6. Ulnar collateral ligament (UCL) injury at the first metacarpophalangeal joint (skier's thumb). Oblique coronal MR image of the thumb shows edema around the torn and retracted UCL (arrow). Note intact radial collateral ligament for comparison (arrowheads).

Ligament and Capsular Injuries

Ligament and capsular injuries in the hand are best characterized using US or MRI (Figure 6-6).[7,8] Injuries at the digits occur due to varus/valgus stress or transient subluxation or dislocation. This commonly occurs at the thumb ("skier's thumb" or "gamekeeper's thumb"). The essential lesion in this condition is tearing of the ulnar collateral ligament (UCL) of the first metacarpophalangeal joint. Imaging may be required for diagnosis of tissue interposed between the torn ligament and bone (Stener lesion). Radiographic stress views may result in interposition of tissue where none was initially present, potentially creating a surgical lesion. Collateral ligaments and capsular structures in other finger joints can also be accurately assessed with US or MRI, with direct visualization of discontinuity.

ARTHRITIS

The articular findings and distribution of joint disease can be best assessed using radiographs (Figure 6-7).[9] However, radiography is insensitive to early erosions and synovitis. MRI

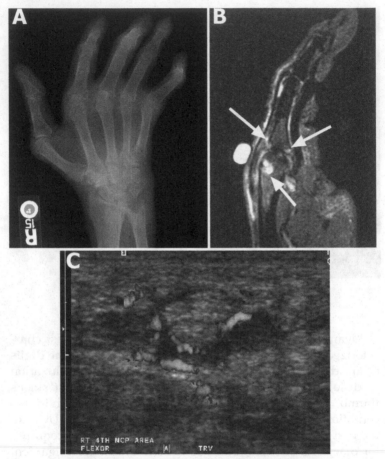

Figure 6-7. Rheumatoid arthritis. (A) AP radiograph of the hand reveals erosions at the wrist and metacarpophalangeal joints with soft tissue swelling and finger deformity characteristic of the disease. (B) Sagittal MR image of a different patient shows synovitis and erosions (arrows) at an MCP joint. (C) Power Doppler US can also be used to demonstrate extent of synovial proliferation (or hyperemia).

is superior for detection of synovial fluid and pannus, tenosynovitis and tendinosis, early bone erosions, and cartilage damage.[9-14] Use of a contrast agent (gadolinium) can help to differentiate between fluid and inflammatory synovial tissue.[10] The quantification of erosions, synovial volume, and vascularity can potentially be used to monitor the response

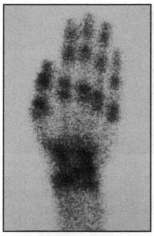

Figure 6-8. Reflex sympathetic dystrophy. Tc-99m-MDP bone scan shows periarticular radiotracer uptake at all joints of the wrist and hand. Bone scan findings in general are nonspecific but can be useful to define multifocality of a pathological process.

to therapy.[15-17] The major drawbacks of MRI as a method for monitoring disease status are its relatively high cost and limited availability. US is a convenient and cost-effective tool for evaluating these findings and can also be used for monitoring treatment response and disease activity, especially if power Doppler is used to assess synovial blood flow.[18]

In patients with polyarthralgia, a whole body bone scan can potentially be useful in order to determine additional articular and entheseal sites of involvement, with subsequent use of radiographs or cross-sectional imaging for correlation. Uptake at enthesial attachment sites (tendon, ligament, or aponeurosis attachment) in extremities suggests psoriatic arthritis or Reiter's disease (reactive arthritis), whereas uptake at enthesial attachments in the spine and pelvis suggest ankylosing spondylitis.

REFLEX SYMPATHETIC DYSTROPHY

When diagnosing reflex sympathetic dystrophy, also known as chronic regional pain syndrome, or Sudeck's Atrophy, radiographs typically show soft-tissue swelling and regional osteoporosis in the absence of significant intra-articular erosion and joint space narrowing. A diffuse increase in periarticular uptake on delayed images can be seen on bone scan (Figure 6-8). However, imaging findings can be nonspecific.[19]

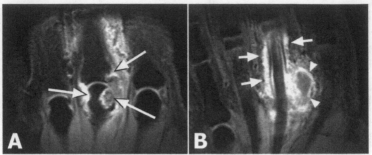

Figure 6-9. Septic arthritis of the hand resulting from a human bite wound. Post-contrast coronal MR images of the hand show erosions (long arrow) at the third metacarpophalangeal joint associated with enhancing septic tenosynovitis (short arrows) and adjacent abscess (arrow).

INFECTION

Radiography can provide initial assessment of suspected infection; it is also useful as a convenient tool for follow-up after treatment. However, radiographs are insensitive in early stages and cannot determine the extent of soft tissue involvement. Nuclear medicine scanning is sensitive but lacks specificity and is limited with regard to extent and soft tissue disease.[20] US can be used for detection of soft tissue abscesses, which appear as focal fluid collections, with the differential diagnosis narrowed by the appropriate clinical context[21]; however, detection of a fluid collection alone is nonspecific. Debris may be seen in the dependent portion of the collection, and the indistinct margin of abscesses and hyperemia on Doppler may allow differentiation from ganglion cysts. The absence of joint fluid virtually excludes septic arthritis unless there is active drainage through a skin ulcer. Septic tenosynovitis can also be detected. Furthermore, US can be used to guide aspiration of fluid collections.

MRI is excellent for identifying the extent of infection in bone and soft tissue as well as fluid collections and tendon involvement. The presence of joint effusion and synovial thickening would suggest the diagnosis of septic arthritis; however, other inflammatory arthropathies can appear identical, so clinical correlation is important.[11] Bone marrow edema and abnormal enhancement in this context suggest the diagnosis of osteomyelitis (Figure 6-9).

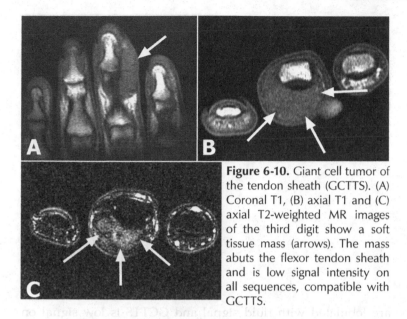

Figure 6-10. Giant cell tumor of the tendon sheath (GCTTS). (A) Coronal T1, (B) axial T1 and (C) axial T2-weighted MR images of the third digit show a soft tissue mass (arrows). The mass abuts the flexor tendon sheath and is low signal intensity on all sequences, compatible with GCTTS.

In the hand, implantation of infection via human bite or a punch to the mouth is a common scenario, typically occurring at the dorsum of a metacarpophalangeal joint. Radiography can demonstrate fractures, tooth fragments, and other foreign bodies. Infectious tenosynovitis, osteomyelitis, and septic arthritis caused predominantly by *Staphylococcus aureus* or *S. pyogenes* are known complications. Extent of infection is best evaluated with MRI.[22,23]

SOFT TISSUE MASSES

As with the wrist, most soft tissue mass-like lesions in the hand are benign.[24-29] Ganglion cysts are particularly prevalent, especially around the joints and tendon sheaths. The major clinical differential in patients with palpable masses along the flexor tendons of the fingers is giant cell tumor of the tendon sheath (GCTTS) (Figure 6-10) and ganglion cyst. On US, ganglia appear cystic without Doppler flow, while GCTTS is solid, hypoechoic, vascular, and adjacent to the flexor tendon. MRI can accurately characterize lesions as well; ganglion cysts

Figure 6-11. Fracture through an enchondroma. Radiograph of the hand shows pathological fracture through a lytic lesion in the first metacarpal. Note curvilinear calcifications within the lesion characteristic of chondroid matrix.

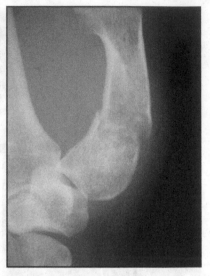

are lobulated with fluid signal and GCTTS is low signal on all sequences. Vascular malformations and lipomas are other common benign entities. MR angiography of the hand can be used to create an arterial "road map" prior to surgery in case of vascular malformations. Similar to other areas of the body, sarcomas are important to exclude; a solid or heterogeneous lesion without definitive benign features should be considered for biopsy.

BONE TUMOR

Radiographs are the first line of investigation when bone tumor is suspected. Enchondroma (Figure 6-11) is the most common bone tumor seen in the hand[30]; radiographic findings of a well-defined, lobulated medullary lesion with small foci of curvilinear calcifications can be diagnostic in most cases. Aggressive features of a bone lesion include cortical breakthrough; associated soft tissue mass; periosteal reaction; and lack of a thin, sclerotic margin. Presentation with pain should raise the suspicion of fracture or malignant nature. Expansion or endosteal scalloping can be a benign feature, but scalloping greater than two-thirds the normal thickness of the

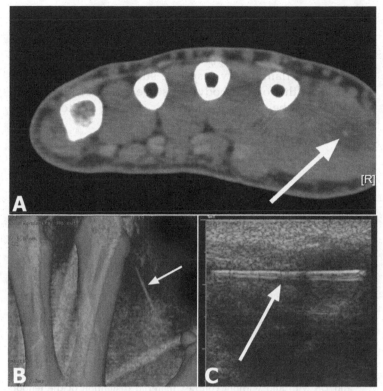

Figure 6-12. Foreign body. (A) CT of the hand reveals a tiny hyperdense focus at first webspace (arrow), corresponding to a splinter not seen on radiographs. (B) 3-Dimensional reformatted CT with color rendering shows capability of this modality for advanced image processing facilitating interventional planning. (C) US is especially advantageous for detection of foreign bodies. Note linear echogenic nature of the splinter (arrow) using this modality.

long bone cortex is a relatively aggressive sign. MRI can be ordered to demonstrate the intramedullary extent of tumor as well as the presence of any soft tissue extension. Whole body bone scan is reserved for detection of metastatic lesions in the proper clinical context.

FOREIGN BODY

Initial assessment should begin with radiographs. Glass and metals can usually be readily seen. However, not all foreign bodies are radio-opaque (Figure 6-12). US can be employed as the next line of investigation. The foreign body is usually echogenic; however, if located inside an echogenic structure such as a tendon, it can be hard to visualize. The presence of inflammatory response such as hypoechoic rim surrounding the foreign body can serve as a secondary sign. MR or CT can be used if radiographs and US fail to demonstrate the finding.[31]

REFERENCES

1. Tagliafico A, Rubino M, Autuori A, Bianchi S, Martinoli C. Wrist and hand ultrasound. *Semin Musculoskelet Radiol*. 2007;11(2):95-104.

2. Bencardino JT. MR imaging of tendon lesions of the hand and wrist. *Magn Reson Imaging Clin N Am*. 2004;12(2):333-347.

3. Clavero JA, Golano P, Farinas O, Alomar X, Monill JM, Esplugas M. Extensor mechanism of the fingers: MR imaging–anatomic correlation. *RadioGraphics*. 2003; 23:593–611.

4. Adler RS, Finzel KC. The complementary roles of MR imaging and ultrasound of tendons. *Radiol Clin North Am*. 2005;43(4):771-807.

5. Parellada JA, Balkissoon AR, Hayes CW, Conway WF. Bowstring injury of the flexor tendon pulley system: MR imaging. *AJR Am J Roentgenol*. 1996;167(2):347-349.

6. Hauger O, Chung CB, Lektrakul N, et al. Pulley system in the fingers: normal anatomy and simulated lesions in cadavers at MR imaging, CT, and US with and without contrast material distention of the tendon sheath. *Radiology*. 2000;217(1):201-212.

7. Clavero JA, Alomar X, Monill JM, et al. MR imaging of ligament and tendon injuries of the fingers. *RadioGraphics*. 2002;22(2):237-256.

8. Ebrahim FS, De Maeseneer M, Jager T, Marcelis S, Jamadar DA, Jacobson JA. Tears of the thumb and Stener lesions: technique, pattern based approach, and differential diagnosis. *RadioGraphics*. 2006; 26:1007–1020.

9. Clement JP 4th, Kassarjian A, Palmer WE. Synovial inflammatory processes in the hand. *Eur J Radiol*. 2005;56(3):307-318.

10. Jevtic V, Watt I, Rozman B, et al. Precontrast and postcontrast (Gd-DTPA) magnetic resonance imaging of hand joints in patients with rheumatoid arthritis. *Clin Radiol*. 1993;48(3):176-181.

11. Jbara M, Patnana M, Kazmi F, Beltran J. MR imaging: arthropathies and infectious conditions of the elbow, wrist, and hand. *Magn Reson Imaging Clin N Am*. 2004;12(2):361-379.

12. Farrant JM, O'Connor PJ, Grainger AJ. Advanced imaging in rheumatoid arthritis. Part 1: synovitis. *Skeletal Radiol*. 2007;36(5):381-389.

13. Farrant JM, Grainger AJ, O'Connor PJ. Advanced imaging in rheumatoid arthritis: part 2: erosions. *Skeletal Radiol*. 2007;36(4):269-279.

14. Taouli B, Zaim S, Peterfy CG, et al. Rheumatoid Arthritis of the Hand and Wrist: Comparison of Three Imaging Techniques. *AJR Am J Roentgenol*. 2004;182(4):937-943.

15. Klarlund M, Ostergaard M, Jensen KE, et al. Magnetic resonance imaging of the wrist in early rheumatoid arthritis reveals a high prevalence of erosions at four months after symptom onset. *Ann Rheum Dis.* 1998;57:350–356.

16. Savnik A, Malmskov H, Thomsen HS, et al. MRI of the wrist and finger joints in inflammatory joint diseases at 1-year interval: MRI features to predict bone erosions. *Eur Radiol.* 2002;12:1203–1210.

17. Lorenzen I. Magnetic resonance imaging, radiography, and scintigraphy of the finger joints: one year follow up of patients with early arthritis—the TIRA group. *Ann Rheum Dis.* 2000;59:521–528.

18. Kamishima T, Tanimura K, Henmi M, et al. Power Doppler ultrasound of rheumatoid synovitis: quantification of vascular signal and analysis of interobserver variability. *Skeletal Radiol.* 2009;38(5):467-72.

19. Schürmann M, Zaspel J, Löhr P, et al. Imaging in early posttraumatic complex regional pain syndrome: a comparison of diagnostic methods. *Clin J Pain.* 2007;23(5):449-457.

20. Prandini N, Lazzeri E, Rossi B, Erba P, Parisella MG, Signore A. Nuclear medicine imaging of bone infections. *Nucl Med Commun.* 2006;27(8):633-644.

21. Bureau NJ, Chhem RK, Cardinal E. Musculoskeletal infections: US manifestations. *RadioGraphics.* 1999;19:1585-1592.

22. Pineda C, Vargas A, Rodríguez AV. Imaging of osteomyelitis: current concepts. *Infect Dis Clin North Am.* 2006;20(4):789-825.

23. Santiago Restrepo C, Giménez CR, McCarthy K. Imaging of osteomyelitis and musculoskeletal soft tissue infections: current concepts. *Rheum Dis Clin North Am.* 2003;29(1):89-109.

24. Wu JS, Hochman MG. Soft-tissue tumors and tumorlike lesions: a systematic imaging approach. *Radiology.* 2009;253(2):297-316.

25. Middleton WD, Patel V, Teefey SA, Boyer MI. Giant cell tumors of the tendon sheath: analysis of sonographic findings. *AJR Am J Roentgenol.* 2004;183(2):337-339.

26. Horcajadas AB, Lafuente JL, de la Cruz Burgos R, et al. Ultrasound and MR findings in tumor and tumor-like lesions of the fingers. *Eur Radiol.* 2003;13(4):672-685.

27. Connell DA, Koulouris G, Thorn DA, Potter HG. Contrast-enhanced MR angiography of the hand. *RadioGraphics.* 2002;22:583–599.

28. Frassica FJ, Khanna JA, McCarthy EF. The role of MR imaging in soft tissue tumor evaluation: perspective of the orthopedic oncologist and musculoskeletal pathologist. *Magn Reson Imaging Clin N Am.* 2000;8(4):915-927.

29. Kitagawa Y, Ito H, Amano Y, Sawaizumi T, Takeuchi T. MR imaging for preoperative diagnosis and assessment of local tumor extent on localized giant cell tumor of tendon sheath. *Skeletal Radiol.* 2003;32(11):633-638.

30. Peh WC. Digital enchondroma. *Am J Orthop.* 2004;33(8):416.

31. Peterson JJ, Bancroft LW, Kransdorf MJ. Wooden foreign bodies: imaging appearance. *AJR Am J Roentgenol.* 2002;178(3):557-562.

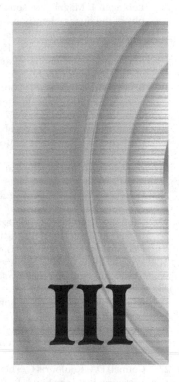

III

*Common
Conditions of the
Elbow, Wrist,
and Hand*

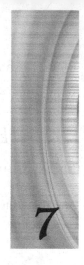

ELBOW INSTABILITY

Min Jung Park, MD, MMSc and Jeffrey Yao, MD

INTRODUCTION

Acute elbow dislocations are relatively common injuries with an average annual incidence of acute dislocation of 6 per 100,000 people.[1] Subsequent elbow instability may be classified based on several criteria, including the chronicity, articulation involved, the direction of displacement of the radial head, the degree of displacement, and the presence or absence of associated fractures (Table 7-1).[2] Historically, elbow trauma and subsequent instability posed significant morbidity to patients,

Culp RW, Jacoby SM. *Musculoskeletal Examination of the Elbow, Wrist, and Hand: Making the Complex Simple* (pp. 139-158). © 2012 Taylor & Francis Group.

Table 7-1

ELBOW INSTABILITY CLASSIFICATION

CRITERIA	PRESENTATION	RADIOGRAPHIC FINDINGS	MANAGEMENT PEARLS
Timing	Acute	Evidence of fractures, frank dislocations, evidence of soft tissue swelling on plain x-rays. AP, lateral, and oblique radiographs should be obtained. When in doubt for incarcerated fragments in the joint, CT scan is recommended.	Ruling out frank fractures and incarcerated intra-articular piece is critical. Careful neurovascular exam should be performed as well as inspection of skin for possible open fracture/dislocation. Closed reduction maneuver should be based on the pattern of dislocation.
	Chronic	With chronic dislocation/subluxation, exam should also start with plain x-rays, then based on history and physical exam, MRI is warranted to evaluate surrounding soft tissue injuries.	Often, closed reduction is difficult or not possible. Patients usually find comfortable position, but not in a functional position. Evaluation should be geared toward obtaining advanced imaging, careful history, and a physical exam to plan possible operative treatment.
	Recurrent	With recurrent dislocations, continuous fluoroscopic exam may be helpful in order to evaluate the range of motion of the elbow and reproduce the symptoms.	With the imaging studies and physical exam, reduction and mode of dislocation should be evaluated to determine the best treatment option based on associated pathologies.

(continued)

Table 7-1 (continued)

ELBOW INSTABILITY CLASSIFICATION

CRITERIA	PRESENTATION	RADIOGRAPHIC FINDINGS	MANAGEMENT PEARLS
Articulation involved	Ulnotrochlear Radioulnar Radio-capitellum	All 3 articulations should be evaluated with plain x-rays, then with CT if incarcerated fracture piece is suspected.	Attempted closed reduction is a key during the acute phase. Immobilization in posterior splint in approximately 30 degrees with the splint extending to the ulnar side of the hand to control supination/pronation is warranted in the setting of fracture or grossly unstable elbow. Stable elbow following closed reduction can be managed in a sling.
Direction of displacement	Valgus Varus Anterior Posterolateral rotatory	Stress radiographs can be useful in diagnosis in these settings (please see Table 7-2).	Direction of displacement is very useful information that can guide us in terms of possible structures involved (eg, MCL in valgus instability).
The degree of displacement	Subluxation dislocation	Although mostly physical exam findings, static radiograph evidence of subluxation can be confirmed on CT.	Patients may be asymptomatic and it is important to evaluate contralateral joint to assess the baseline laxity.

(continued)

Table 7-1 (continued)

ELBOW INSTABILITY CLASSIFICATION

CRITERIA	PRESENTATION	RADIOGRAPHIC FINDINGS	MANAGEMENT PEARLS
Associated fractures	Radial head	Nonspecific findings such as anterior and/or posterior fat pad signs on plain radiographs can be present. CT scan is helpful in the setting of preoperative planning for fractures that meet operative criteria, typically articular step off greater than 2 mm, more than 30% of articular surface involvement, and comminuted fractures.	Supination/pronation should elicit discomfort when there is evidence of fracture. Patients will typically hold their elbow in flexed, pronated position.
	Coronoid	CT scan is almost always warranted in the setting of elbow instability with coronoid fracture to evaluate the stability of MCL.	Based on the extent of the coronoid fracture and the degree of elbow instability, operative management may be warranted (see Table 7-3).
	Olecranon	Most of fractures should be picked up on plain x-rays.	In the setting of elbow instability, the presence of olecranon fracture almost always warrants operative intervention, unless the fracture is nonarticular, only involves the distal tip of the olecranon, or in poor surgical candidate.

as management strategies failed to provide satisfactory results in many instances. Better understanding of the pathoanatomy, early recognition, and intervention for the injuries that lead to elbow instability are critical in achieving good results.

HISTORY

Standard questions such as hand dominance, occupation, mechanism of injury, duration of symptoms, and exacerbating factors should be explored thoroughly. Frequently, the mechanism of injury may lead to the accurate diagnosis of the underlying pathology. Prior surgery for medial or lateral epicondylitis, ulnar nerve surgery, and surgery dealing with the radial head in particular should be explored in detail. In the face of chronic instability, patients typically report recurrent painful clicking, snapping, clunking, or locking of the elbow. The symptoms are reproduced most often during the extension portion of the arc of motion with the forearm in supination.

Most frequently, elbow instability is a result of prior trauma, and patients will provide the inciting injury, such as falling on outstretched hand or receiving a direct blow to the elbow. Even without frank dislocation, any prior elbow trauma should alert examiners to consider elbow instability in the differential diagnosis. Although relatively rare, congenital anatomic variants should also be part of the differential diagnosis, especially if there is no definite history of trauma.

EXAMINATION

An appropriate physical examination serves as a link between the patient's subjective complaints and the pathology of the underlying symptoms (Table 7-2). Prior to the examination of the elbow, it is important to inspect the entire upper extremity, including the cervical spine. Any signs of extrinsic etiology of the elbow pain should be further evaluated when necessary. One should carefully look for prior surgical incisions around the shoulder, forearm, and elbow. Often, physical

Table 7-2

METHODS FOR EXAMINING

EXAMINATION	TECHNIQUE	ILLUSTRATION	POSITIVE FINDING	SIGNIFICANCE
Pivot-shift apprehension test	Supination and valgus moments with axial compression during elbow flexion.	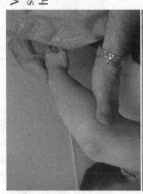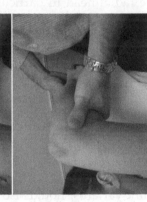	Visible and/or palpable subluxation of radial head.	Degree of radial head displacement can be measured.

(continued)

Table 7-2 (continued)

METHODS FOR EXAMINING

EXAMINATION	TECHNIQUE	ILLUSTRATION	POSITIVE FINDING	SIGNIFICANCE
Posterolateral rotatory drawer test	Similar to Lachman's test of knee, stabilize forearm and humerus and exert gentle pressure on patient's forearm toward the examiner's body.	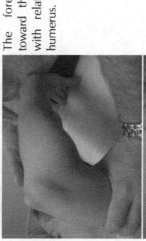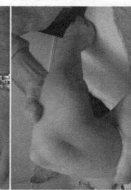	The forearm shifts toward the examiner with relation to the humerus.	Posterolateral rotatory instability.

(continued)

Table 7-2 (continued)

METHODS FOR EXAMINING

EXAMINATION	TECHNIQUE	ILLUSTRATION	POSITIVE FINDING	SIGNIFICANCE
Lift-off test	With their forearm supinated, patients are asked to stand up from the chair, pushing off on the arm support.	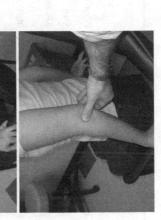	Visible and/or palpable click around the radial head.	Patients may report pain at the lateral elbow with a visible and/or palpable click around the radial head.

(continued)

Table 7-2 (continued)

METHODS FOR EXAMINING

EXAMINATION	TECHNIQUE	ILLUSTRATION	POSITIVE FINDING	SIGNIFICANCE
Tabletop relocation test	With forearm supinated, patents are asked to lean on to the edge of a tabletop, and push down into the table, allowing the elbow to flex.	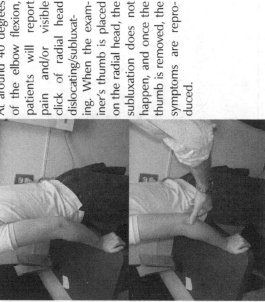	At around 40 degrees of the elbow flexion, patients will report pain and/or visible click of radial head dislocating/subluxating. When the examiner's thumb is placed on the radial head, the subluxation does not happen, and once the thumb is removed, the symptoms are reproduced.	May indicate possible poterolateral rotatory instability of elbow.

(continued)

Table 7-2 (continued)

METHODS FOR EXAMINING

EXAMINATION	TECHNIQUE	ILLUSTRATION	POSITIVE FINDING	SIGNIFICANCE
Stress radiograph of elbow	With the humerus in perfect lateral position, the elbow is flexed slightly at around 30 degrees, with the x-ray cassette placed on the lateral side of the elbow, examiner applies gentle varus or valgus stress on the elbow.	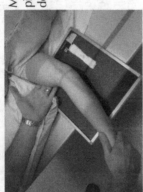	Medial or lateral gapping of the elbow evident on the plain x-ray.	Access varus/valgus instability of the elbow.

exam findings may be subtle, and adequate examination may not be possible due to pain and discomfort.

Typically, patients with elbow instability will localize their pain to the lateral elbow. The typical symptoms of clicking, snapping, clunking, or locking of the elbow occurs more during extension and supination. The most sensitive test for elbow instability is the pivot-shift apprehension test. In Stage I of posterolateral rotatory instability (PLRI), patients may demonstrate a positive pivot-shift test. The pivot-shift test is performed with the patient supine and the arm forward flexed to approximately 120 degrees. Supination and valgus moments with axial compression are applied during elbow flexion (see Table 7-2). In the case of a positive test, the elbow will subluxate maximally at 40 degrees to 70 degrees of flexion.[2] Further flexion will relocate the elbow, and a palpable and visible clunk may be observed. Frequently, frank dislocation and reduction may only be reproduced under anesthesia or following an intra-articular local anesthetic injection. Patients will report discomfort and apprehension during the exam, and the sense of impending dislocation by the patient is interpreted as a positive finding. The posterolateral rotatory drawer test is similar to the Lachman test of the knee. With the shoulder in full external rotation and the arm in overhead position, the examiner holds the forearm as if he or she would hold the leg during the Lachman test. The lateral side of the forearm is rotated away from the humerus, pivoting around the medial collateral ligament so that the radius and ulna subluxate away from the humerus (see Table 7-2).[2] One will often observe a dimple proximal to the radial head as the elbow dislocates. The lift-off test may also reproduce patients' symptoms by having patients attempt to stand up from the sitting position by pushing on the armrests with their hands at the side and the elbow fully supinated (see Table 7-2).[3] With the tabletop test, elevation of the body from the edge of a table with the forearm in supination causes apprehension if elbow instability is present. Lateral elbow support often relieves the apprehension during the test (see Table 7-2).[4] With Stage II instability, the elbow dislocates completely, and the coronoid rests behind the humerus. In Stage IIIa, the anterior band of the medical collateral ligament (MCL) is intact, and the elbow is stable after reduction. Stage IIIb represents a disrupted anterior band of the MCL, and the elbow demonstrates valgus instability. In Stage IIIc, all soft-tissue attachments to the humerus are stripped, and the elbow is grossly unstable even with immobilization.[2] In order to prevent false-positive results with the valgus stress examination, the exam should be performed with the forearm fully pronated. All physical exam findings should be compared with the contralateral side, as some findings may be symmetrical. Valgus and varus instability may be evaluated by using stress radiographs described in the imaging section of this chapter.

PATHOANATOMY

The elbow is divided into a posterior cubital region and an anterior cubital region. The latter region contains the antecubital fossa. The anterior fossa is formed by the brachioradialis laterally and pronator teres medially. The distal biceps tendon divides the antecubital fossa into two halves with the medial half covered by its aponeurotic expansion. The floor of the antecubital fossa is formed by the brachialis muscle. The distal humeral epiphysis is flat and is angled approximately 45 degrees with respect to the humeral shaft. The medial and lateral epicondyles are located outside the articular capsule and provide origins for the collateral ligaments and the flexor/ pronator (medial) and common extensor (lateral) tendons. The elbow is a trocho-ginglymus joint with 2 articulations within one capsule. The trochlea is located medially and articulates with the ulna. Flexion and extension are achieved by the ulnohumeral articulation. The capitellum is separated from the trochlea by a groove. The radiocapitellar and proximal radioulnar articulations provide axial rotation about the elbow. The radial fossa and coronoid fossa accommodate the radial head and coronoid during flexion, and the olecranon fossa accommodates the olecranon during extension. The radiocapitellar and ulnohumeral joints are the common sites of elbow joint instability.

The most common direction of radial head dislocations is posterolateral,[2] and associated fractures significantly increase the likelihood of developing elbow instability and subsequent elbow arthrosis.[5-8] The posterolateral nature of

the displacement is influenced by the coronoid process passing inferior to the trochlea. The ulna tends to supinate along
with the radial head. The MCL complex is composed of anterior, posterior, and transverse segments, of which the anterior
bundle is the most important for elbow stability.[9] The anterior
bundle of the MCL originates from the anteroinferior surface
of the medial epicondyle and inserts on the sublime tubercle
of the coronoid process approximately 18 mm distal to the
tip of the coronoid.[10,11] The lateral collateral ligament (LCL)
complex is made up of the radial collateral ligament, annular
ligament, lateral ulnar collateral ligament, and the accessory
lateral collateral ligament. The LCL originates from the lateral
epicondyle, blends with the annular ligament, and inserts onto
the supinator crest of the proximal ulna. Valgus instability
of the elbow may be chronic (overuse) or post-traumatic in
nature. Post-traumatic valgus instability is often associated
with an MCL injury. Injuries to other soft-tissue structures,
such as common flexor and pronator origin, may also contribute to valgus instability of the elbow. The radial head serves
as a secondary valgus stabilizer of the elbow,[12,13] particularly
when the MCL is deficient. Chronic valgus instability of the
elbow is mainly associated with repeated microtrauma and
attritional rupture of the anterior band of the medial collateral ligament, particularly in throwing athletes.[14] The elbow
is mostly subjected to valgus stress due to its anatomic nature.
Although LCL injuries may lead to varus instability, posterolateral rotatory instability is a more common pattern observed
in the face of LCL injuries.

Proximal radioulnar joint (PRUJ) dislocations are associated
with Monteggia fracture-dislocation patterns with a history
of trauma and a proximal ulna fracture. The injury pattern
can be classified based on the Bado classification, where the
fracture dislocation is classified based on the direction of the
radial head dislocation, with Type I anterior, Type II posterior,
Type III lateral, and Type IV with an associated proximal
radius fracture (Table 7-3).[15] Type II can be further subdivided
with Type IIa with a distal olecranon and coronoid fracture,
Type IIb with a meta-diaphyseal junction fracture of ulna,
Type IIc with a diaphyseal ulnar fracture, and Type IId with
fracture extension to the proximal half of the ulna.[16]

Table 7-3

BADO CLASSIFICATION OF MONTEGGIA FRACTURE-DISLOCATIONS

TYPE	DESCRIPTION
I	Anterior dislocation of the radial head
II	Posterior dislocation of the radial head
III	Lateral dislocation of the radial head
IV	Fracture of the proximal radius and ulna with dislocation of the radial head

With its role as insertion point of the MCL and anterior buttress of the ulna, the coronoid plays a key role in elbow stability as well. Coronoid fractures are classified based on the size of the fracture fragment.[17] Type I is a simple avulsion at the tip of the coronoid, Type II involves approximately 50% of the coronoid, and Type III represents fracture involving greater than 50% of articulation. O'Driscoll and colleagues modified the classification. The Type I pattern is transverse fracture of the tip of the coronoid with subclassification based on the size of the fragment either greater or smaller than 2 mm; Type II is the pattern involving anteromedial facet of the coronoid process with the subtypes based on associated fracture of the tip, or sublime tubercle; and Type III is the pattern where coronoid fracture is at the base with subtypes based on location of the body fracture, either coronoid body and base, or transolecranon basal coronoid fracture (Table 7-4).[18] Surgical options for coronoid fractures depend on the size of the displaced fragment. With a relatively small tip avulsion, a lasso repair of the anterior capsule may be successful. For a larger fragment, screw fixation from posterior ulnar or anteromedial plate fixation may provide adequate fixation.

The term *terrible triad* refers to an elbow dislocation along with fracture of the radial head and a coronoid fracture. As described previously, the 2 structures play key roles in elbow stability, and the terrible triad injury often leads to recurrent

Table 7-4

O'DRISCOLL CLASSIFICATION OF CORONOID FRACTURES

CLASSIFICATION	DESCRIPTION	SUBTYPES
Type I	Tip of coronoid	Tip > 2 mm
		Tip < 2 mm
Type II	Anteromedial coronoid	Anteromedial only
		Anteromedial with tip fracture
		Anteromedial with tip and sublime tubercle
Type III	Base of coronoid	Coronoid body
		Transolecranon

instability and subsequent arthritis. The posterior Monteggia variant consists of posterior radial head dislocation along with a proximal ulna fracture and coronoid fracture. This pattern of injury is described mainly in older women who suffer low-energy trauma. On the contrary, the radius and ulna are displaced anteriorly in a transolecranon fracture-dislocation. Often, the proximal radioulnar joint is maintained.[19] Transolecranon fracture dislocations are often a result of a high-energy trauma. Although relatively rare, the injury pattern is associated with anterior instability of the elbow.[20]

IMAGING

As an initial assessment of elbow instability, standard radiograph views including posteroanterior (PA), lateral, and oblique views should be obtained. Radiographs will allow one to assess the alignment of ulnohumeral, radio-humeral, and radioulnar articulations. Any signs of subtle fractures should be identified, and when in doubt, a CT scan should be obtained to assess any subtle fractures or incarcerated fragments. Often, lateral stress radiographs may show the rotator subluxation of the radial head. The stress radiograph is obtained with the lateral side of the elbow against the x-ray plate with the shoulder and wrist in the same plane as the elbow, then directing the x-ray beam from medial to lateral (see Table 7-2). A lateral stress radiograph at the point of maximum rotatory subluxation during the pivot shift test may be helpful as well. Continuous imaging with image intensifier may also help discern any dynamic nature of the instability.

TREATMENT

In the acute setting, a careful neurovascular exam must be performed, and the skin should be examined to rule out an open fracture-dislocation. An initial reduction attempt should be made under adequate sedation. The typical reduction maneuver involves axial traction followed by supination and flexion of the elbow. If stable reduction is achieved, closed treatment is sufficient. Immobilization for 1 week in a posterior splint followed by early range-of-motion exercises is instituted. Follow-up radiographs are obtained at the 1-week visit and as needed during rehabilitation.

With chronic elbow instability, many patients will require some form of surgical treatment to regain joint stability. Lateral collateral ligament complex injury should be properly assessed and repaired. The LCL repair using graft is the generally accepted treatment of choice, and the ligament reconstruction entails passing the auto- or allograft through a bone tunnel from the lateral humeral epicondyle to the supinator crest of the ulna with fixation achieved by either suture anchors or interference screws. Palmaris longus, triceps fascia, semitendinosus, gracilis, plantaris, and Achilles grafts are reported to be used to reconstruct the LCL.[21-27] If MCL is intact, LCL should be repaired with the forearm pronated. However, if MCL injury is suspected, LCL should be repaired with the forearm in supination in order to prevent medial opening from over-tightening lateral repair. The MCL repair is indicated if the elbow is unstable after LCL repair, proper assessment, and/or fixation of the coronoid and radial head.[28]

In most cases, surgical management is indicated if there is radial head fracture associated with elbow instability. Radial head replacement is recommended in the case of comminution with more than 3 fragments, while internal fixation with small compression screws yields good results in simple fractures.[29-33] Even in the case of a comminuted radial head fracture, internal fixation tends to produce better results compared to radial head excision.[34] In fact, radial head resection is often a source of elbow pain and posterolateral instability and is rarely indicated currently.[35] If there is coronoid fracture along with radial head fracture, ligament reconstruction is often needed in addition to internal fixation. Most coronoid fractures should be surgically addressed in the setting of elbow instability.[36,37] In some instances of severe chronic instability with or without evidence of post-traumatic arthritis, total elbow arthroplasty may be the only option. Chronic unreduced dislocations and recurrent instability in complex injuries are very difficult to manage. In addition to surgical intervention, they often require the use of a hinged external fixator to hold the elbow in a reduced position.[38-40] For terrible triad injuries involving elbow dislocations along with a coronoid fracture and radial head fracture, either radial head fixation or replacement along with coronoid fixation are required to achieve satisfactory results. The LCL and/or MCL may need to be repaired as well if the elbow is not stable enough after radial head and coronoid fixation. A hinged external fixator can be used with an unstable elbow with fracture fixation and ligament reconstruction.[28,36] In the posterior Monteggia variant injuries, recognition of coronoid and surgical fixation is the key to achieving a good result.[16,41] Transolecranon fracture-dislocations require posterior plate fixation of the olecranon. Careful examination of coronoid is warranted in this case as Type III coronoid fractures are frequently associated with the injury pattern. The collateral ligaments and radial head are intact in most of these injuries.

CONCLUSION

The elbow is an unforgiving joint. With 3 complex articulations and elaborate soft-tissues stabilizers, it is easy to miss injuries associated with acute trauma or chronic instability. It is important to recognize associated radial head or coronoid fractures in the face of an acute dislocation. Careful evaluation of the MCL and the LCL is needed to guide the appropriate surgical strategy. Patients should be well-informed regarding the prognosis of such injuries and have appropriate expectations following surgery. The use of hinged external fixators in addition to surgical procedures should be considered in all cases with elbow instability.

ACKNOWLEDGMENT

Dr. Min Jung Park would like to thank Drs. Chancellor Gray and Mara Schenker for their help with the preparation of this chapter.

REFERENCES

1. Linscheid RL, Wheeler DK. Elbow dislocations. *JAMA*. 1965;194(11):1171-1176.
2. O'Driscoll SW. Classification and evaluation of recurrent instability of the elbow. *Clin Ortho Rel Res*. 2000;370:34-43.
3. Regan W, Lapner PC. Prospective evaluation of two diagnostic apprehension signs for posterolateral instability of the elbow. *J Shoulder Elbow Surg*. 2006;15(3):344-346.
4. Arvind CH, Hargreaves DG. Tabletop relocation test: a new clinical test for posterolateral rotatory instability of the elbow. *J Shoulder Elbow Surg*. 2006;15(6):707-708.
5. Broberg MA, Morrey BF. Results of treatment of fracture-dislocations of the elbow. *Clin Ortho Rel Res*. 1987;216:109-119.
6. Josefsson PO, Gentz CF, Johnell O, Wendeberg B. Dislocations of the elbow and intraarticular fractures. *Clin Ortho Rel Res*. 1989;246:126-130.
7. Nestor BJ, O'Driscoll SW, Morrey BF. Ligamentous reconstruction for posterolateral rotatory instability of the elbow. *J Bone Joint Surg*. 1992;74(8):1235-1241.
8. O'Driscoll SW. Elbow instability. *Hand Clinics*. 1994;10(3):405-415.
9. Floris S, Olsen BS, Dalstra M, Sojbjerg JO, Sneppen O. The medial collateral ligament of the elbow joint: anatomy and kinematics. *J Shoulder Elbow Surg*. 1998;7(4):345-351.
10. Cage DJ, Abrams RA, Callahan JJ, Botte MJ. Soft tissue attachments of the ulnar coronoid process. An anatomic study with radiographic correlation. *Clin Ortho Rel Res*. 1995;320:154-158.
11. O'Driscoll SW, Jaloszynski R, Morrey BF, An KN. Origin of the medial ulnar collateral ligament. *J Hand Surg*. 1992;17(1):164-168.
12. Deutch SR, Jensen SL, Tyrdal S, Olsen BS, Sneppen O. Elbow joint stability following experimental osteoligamentous injury and reconstruction. *J Shoulder Elbow Surg*. 2003;12(5):466-471.

13. Jensen SL, Deutch SR, Olsen BS, Sojbjerg JO, Sneppen O. Laxity of the elbow after experimental excision of the radial head and division of the medial collateral ligament. Efficacy of ligament repair and radial head prosthetic replacement: a cadaver study. *J Bone Joint Surg Br.* 2003;85(7):1006-1010.

14. Jobe FW, Stark H, Lombardo SJ. Reconstruction of the ulnar collateral ligament in athletes. *J Bone Joint Surg.* 1986;68(8):1158-1163.

15. Bado JL. The Monteggia lesion. *Clin Ortho Rel Res.* 1967;50:71-86.

16. Jupiter JB, Leibovic SJ, Ribbans W, Wilk RM. The posterior Monteggia lesion. *J Ortho Trauma.* 1991;5(4):395-402.

17. Regan W, Morrey B. Fractures of the coronoid process of the ulna. *J Bone Joint Surg.* 1989;71(9):1348-1354.

18. O'Driscoll SW, Jupiter JB, Cohen MS, Ring D, McKee MD. Difficult elbow fractures: pearls and pitfalls. *Instr Course Lectures.* 2003;52:113-134.

19. Ring D, Jupiter JB, Sanders RW, Mast J, Simpson NS. Transolecranon fracture-dislocation of the elbow. *J Ortho Trauma.* 1997;11(8):545-550.

20. Torchia ME, DiGiovine NM. Anterior dislocation of the elbow in an arm wrestler. *J Shoulder Elbow Surg.* 1998;7(5):539-541.

21. Eygendaal D. Ligamentous reconstruction around the elbow using triceps tendon. *Acta Orthopaedica Scandinavica.* 2004;75(5):516-523.

22. Lee BP, Teo LH. Surgical reconstruction for posterolateral rotatory instability of the elbow. *J Shoulder Elbow Surg.* 2003;12(5):476-479.

23. Olsen BS, Sojbjerg JO. The treatment of recurrent posterolateral instability of the elbow. *J Bone Joint Surg Br.* 2003;85(3):342-346.

24. Rizio L. Lateral ulnar collateral ligament reconstruction in a skeletally immature patient. *Am J Sports Med.* 2005;33(3):439-442.

25. Sanchez-Sotelo J, Morrey BF, O'Driscoll SW. Ligamentous repair and reconstruction for posterolateral rotatory instability of the elbow. *J Bone Joint Surg Br.* 2005;87(1):54-61.

26. Cohen MS. Lateral collateral ligament instability of the elbow. *Hand Clinics.* 2008;24(1):69-77.

27. Paterson R, Cohen B, Taylor D, Bourne A, Black J. Reconstruction of the lateral ligaments of the ankle using semi-tendinosis graft. *Foot Ankle International.* 2000;21(5):413-419.

28. Mathew PK, Athwal GS, King GJ. Terrible triad injury of the elbow: current concepts. *JAAOS.* 2009;17(3):137-151.

29. Ashwood N, Bain GI, Unni R. Management of Mason type-III radial head fractures with a titanium prosthesis, ligament repair, and early mobilization. *J Bone Joint Surg.* 2004;86-A(2):274-280.

30. Ikeda M, Yamashina Y, Kamimoto M, Oka Y. Open reduction and internal fixation of comminuted fractures of the radial head using low-profile mini-plates. *J Bone Joint Surg Br.* 2003;85(7):1040-1044.

31. Ring D, Quintero J, Jupiter JB. Open reduction and internal fixation of fractures of the radial head. *J Bone Joint Surg.* 2002;84-A(10):1811-1815.

32. Ring D. Open reduction and internal fixation of fractures of the radial head. *Hand Clinics.* 2004;20(4):415-427, vi.

33. Ring D. Displaced, unstable fractures of the radial head: fixation vs. replacement—what is the evidence? *Injury.* 2008;39(12):1329-1337.

34. Ikeda M, Sugiyama K, Kang C, Takagaki T, Oka Y. Comminuted fractures of the radial head: comparison of resection and internal fixation. Surgical technique. *J Bone Joint Surg.* 2006;88 Suppl 1 Pt 1:11-23.
35. Hall JA, McKee MD. Posterolateral rotatory instability of the elbow following radial head resection. *J Bone Joint Surg.* 2005;87(7):1571-1579.
36. Pugh DM, Wild LM, Schemitsch EH, King GJ, McKee MD. Standard surgical protocol to treat elbow dislocations with radial head and coronoid fractures. *J Bone Joint Surg.* 2004;86-A(6):1122-1130.
37. Ring D, Jupiter JB, Zilberfarb J. Posterior dislocation of the elbow with fractures of the radial head and coronoid. *J Bone Joint Surg.* 2002;84-A(4):547-551.
38. Jupiter JB, Ring D. Treatment of unreduced elbow dislocations with hinged external fixation. *J Bone Joint Surg.* 2002;84-A(9):1630-1635.
39. McKee MD, Bowden SH, King GJ, et al. Management of recurrent, complex instability of the elbow with a hinged external fixator. *J Bone Joint Surg Br.* 1998;80(6):1031-1036.
40. Ruch DS, Triepel CR. Hinged elbow fixation for recurrent instability following fracture dislocation. *Injury.* 2001;32 Suppl 4:SD70-D78.
41. Ring D, Jupiter JB, Simpson NS. Monteggia fractures in adults. *J Bone Joint Surg.* 1998;80(12):1733-1744.

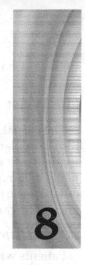

8

LIGAMENT INJURIES
OF THE
WRIST AND HAND

Danielle Scher, MD and Jennifer Moriatis Wolf, MD

INTRODUCTION

Wrist and hand ligament injuries are common. These injuries are often under-recognized in the acute setting, especially in cases of polytrauma, and patients may have delayed presentation with pain and disability. This chapter will focus on some of the most common ligament injuries found in the wrist and the hand, with recommendations for imaging, diagnosis, and treatment.

Culp RW, Jacoby SM. *Musculoskeletal Examination of the Elbow, Wrist, and Hand: Making the Complex Simple* (pp. 159-182). © 2012 Taylor & Francis Group.

The Wrist

The carpal ligaments can be divided into intracapsular and intra-articular with intracapsular ligaments being further subdivided into extrinsic and intrinsic ligaments. Extrinsic ligaments originate within the forearm crossing the wrist joint, and intrinsic ligaments are those that both originate and insert among the carpal bones.

History

Patients with ligamentous injuries of the wrist may present after an acute injury or with a history of untreated sprain with later development of chronic hand or wrist pain and deformity. Acute carpal instability can be either direct (ie, a crush or blast injury causing a global disruption of the carpus)[1] or indirect (ie, a result of extension, ulnar deviation, and intercarpal supination).[2] Perilunate dislocations represent a high-energy carpal injury that may occur after a fall from height or motor vehicle crash. These are the most severe injuries to the ligaments and bones of the carpus, often involving disruption of the scapholunate (SL), lunotriquetral (LT), and several volar radiocarpal ligaments.

Patients presenting with SL dissociation can present after a fall onto their outstretched hand, a fall backwards onto the hand,[3] or after an iatrogenic injury sustained during a dorsal ganglion excision.[4,5] These patients commonly report weakness in grip, giving way, a snap or click during use, and pain and local tenderness over the torn ligament in the acute injury.[3,6] LT dissociation may present after an axial loading injury onto the extended wrist.[7] Pain is reported with pronation and supination against resistance,[7] and patients often describe weakness or instability.[8]

In palmar midcarpal instability, patients will describe a painful clunk when they pronate the wrist with ulnar deviation.[9] In contrast, patients with radial midcarpal instability, secondary to rotatory subluxation of the scaphoid, present with pain and tenderness over the dorsal aspect of the wrist.

Traumatic triangular fibrocartilage complex (TFCC) tears can occur secondary to either the patient falling on a fixed outstretched hand with his or her rotating body causing a hyperpronation injury, dorsal dislocation, or a hypersupination injury, volar dislocation, or having his or her hand caught in a rotating machine.[10] Up to 60% of distal radius fractures are associated with a TFCC tear.[11]

Examination

A key portion in the ligamentous examination of the wrist is the testing of the contralateral side in every patient in order to determine his or her normal level of laxity.

Acute carpal ligament injuries typically present with moderate swelling, ecchymosis, abrasions, and areas of point tenderness that can be indicative of the primary location of the abnormality.[12] In acute injuries, range of motion is usually limited by pain, whereas range of motion tends to normalize with chronic injuries. Injury to median or ulnar nerves may be secondary to the initial traumatic event, compression by the dislocated bones or soft-tissue swelling, and therefore a thorough neurovascular exam should be performed and documented.

When a SL ligament tear is suspected, the pathologic instability of the scaphoid can be assessed using the Watson's/scaphoid shift test (Table 8-1). In this provocative test, the examiner's thumb opposes the normal rotation of the scaphoid during radial deviation, and in a patient with ligamentous laxity, the scaphoid may be forced out of its fossa only to return to its normal position with a painful "clunk" as the wrist is brought into ulnar deviation.[13]

Dorsal pain at the SL interval, while not specific, can represent a partial SL tear versus a ganglion or capsular injury. Another provocative test for determining an SL injury is the SL ballottement test, which stabilizes the lunate while displacing the scaphoid dorsally and palmarly.

A positive midcarpal shift test, when a painful click is reproduced with axial compression, ulnar deviation, and pronation of the hand on the forearm are indicative of palmar midcarpal instability (see Table 8-1).[14] Patients with radial midcarpal instability can display a "catch-up clunk," pain in the scaphoid region with resisted finger extension, and a positive Watson's/scaphoid shift test.[9]

The ulnar fovea sign is a highly sensitive and specific test for determining foveal disruption of the distal radioulnar ligaments and ulnotriquetral ligament injuries (see Table 8-1).

Methods for Examination

Table 8-1

EXAMINATION	TECHNIQUE	ILLUSTRATION	GRADING SYSTEM	SIGNIFICANCE
Wrist				
Watson's/Scaphoid shift test	With the patient seated, place the elbow flat on the table with the forearm in neutral and the wrist elevated perpendicular to the table. The examiner's thumb is placed at the volar scaphoid tubercle, with the index finger on the proximal pole and distal radial articular surface dorsally. The wrist is brought from ulnar to radial deviation while axially loading the wrist and pushing the scaphoid dorsally with the thumb. A positive test is a painful clunk as the scaphoid subluxes over the rim of the radius.	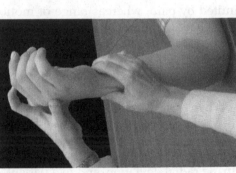		Indicates scapholunate instability secondary to a tear of the scapholunate interosseous ligament.

(continued)

Table 8-1 (continued)

Methods for Examination

EXAMINATION	TECHNIQUE	ILLUSTRATION	GRADING SYSTEM	SIGNIFICANCE
Lunotriquetral shuck test	With the patient positioned similarly to the scaphoid shift test, the examiner places one hand holding the lunate volarly and dorsally, places the other hand on the triquetrum, and attempts to shift them by pushing with one hand and pulling with the other. A positive test elicits pain and crepitance or motion.	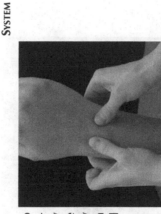		Indicates lunotriquetral injury or tear.

(continued)

Table 8-1 (continued)

Methods for Examination

EXAMINATION	TECHNIQUE	ILLUSTRATION	GRADING SYSTEM	SIGNIFICANCE
Ulnar fovea test	With the arm positioned on an examination table, the examiner grasps the wrist and places the index or middle finger to find the foveal recess just above and volar to the tip of the ulnar styloid, above the flexor carpi ulnaris tendon. Firm pressure within this "soft spot" reproduces pain in the patient complaining of ulnar-sided pain.	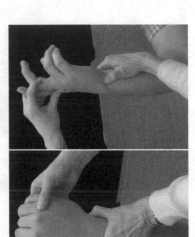		Indicates injury to the ulnotriquetral ligaments or foveal disruption of the distal radioulnar joint (DRU).

(continued)

Table 8-1 (continued)

Methods for Examination

EXAMINATION	TECHNIQUE	ILLUSTRATION	GRADING SYSTEM	SIGNIFICANCE
Lichtman midcarpal shift test	The examiner stabilizes the forearm with one hand, holding the subject's wrist pronated. The examiner's thumb is positioned over the dorsal distal capitate region of the patient's wrist while grasping the wrist and attempting to push the wrist volarly. The wrist is ulnarly deviated while maintaining volarly directed pressure. If the wrist clunks as it moves into ulnar deviation, this is a positive test.	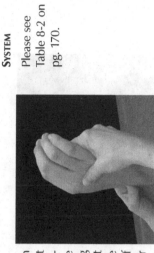	Please see Table 8-2 on pg. 170.	Indicates midcarpal instability and severity of instability if present.

(continued)

Table 8-1 (continued)

Methods for Examination

EXAMINATION	TECHNIQUE	ILLUSTRATION	GRADING SYSTEM	SIGNIFICANCE
DRUJ piano key test	The examiner stabilizes the radius with one hand and grips the ulna with the other and attempts to push it up and down like a piano key.	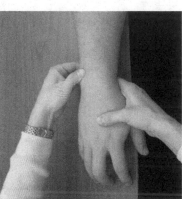		Indicates DRUJ instability.
Ulnocarpal stress test	With the upper arm on an examination table and the forearm held perpendicular to the examination table, the examiner axially loads the wrist while bringing it into ulnar deviation; a positive test reproduces the pain the patient experiences.			Indicates possible ulnocarpal impaction or TFCC tears.

(continued)

Table 8-1 (continued)

Methods for Examination

Examination	Technique	Illustration	Grading System	Significance
Hand				
Proximal interphalangeal joint stress exam	The examiner stabilizes the proximal phalanx with the nondominant hand and grasps the middle phalanx with the other hand, moving it in the radial and ulnar directions with the joint at 0 and 30 degrees.	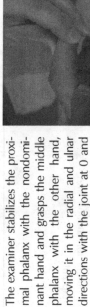		Motion or clunking, particularly with the joint in full extension, indicates injury to the collateral ligaments.
Thumb MCP stress exam (collateral ligament stress exam)	While stabilizing the metacarpal shaft, the examiner applies a radial stress by moving the proximal phalanx radially at 0 and 40 degrees flexion. This is repeated in the ulnar direction.	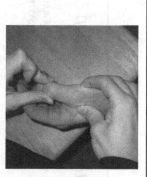		If the examination causes pain but the patient has a definite endpoint, it indicates a partial collateral ligament tear. Absence of an endpoint on stress examination is highly suspicious for a complete collateral ligament tear.

(continued)

Table 8-1 (continued)

Methods for Examination

EXAMINATION	TECHNIQUE	ILLUSTRATION	GRADING SYSTEM	SIGNIFICANCE
Other MCP stress exam	The examiner flexes the MCP joint of interest to 90 degrees, then moves the finger radially and ulnarly and compares it to others for motion and endpoint.			If the finger has a painful arc at 90 degrees or does not have an endpoint, the patient may have a sprain or complete tear of the collateral ligament of the MCP joint

Table 8-2

GRADING SYSTEM FOR THE
LICHTMAN MIDCARPAL SHIFT TEST

GRADE	MIDCARPAL TRANSLATION	CLUNK
I	None	None
II	Minimal	Minimal
III	Moderate	Moderate
IV	Maximal	Significant
V	Self-induced	Self-induced

This provocative test is positive when the patient reports that the tenderness felt on exam has the same quality as the pain that he or she had been experiencing.[15] Distal radioulnar joint (DRUJ) injuries may be assessed with the table press test, ulnar-sided wrist pain elicited when the patients use a table to push themselves up from a seated position, and the piano key test, pain and crepitus elicited when the radius is stabilized and the ulna is translated in an anteroposterior direction (see Table 8-1).[12]

Patients with a TFCC injury display tenderness to palpation in the soft depression between the pisiform and ulnar styloid.[16] The ulnocarpal stress test can be used to detect disk tears with the elbow held at 90 degrees and the wrist held in maximum ulnar deviation. The examiner then applies an axial load through the wrist while bringing the wrist through passive pronation-supination.[17] A positive test is indicated by the production of ulnar-sided wrist pain.

Pathoanatomy

Perilunate instability is secondary to a disruption of intrinsic carpal ligaments generally leading to instability between the proximal carpal row, with lunate dislocation as the final injury.[9] In contrast, laxity of the extrinsic carpal ligaments and associated carpal subluxation is defined as midcarpal instability.[9] This is commonly seen in younger females.[18]

The proximal carpal row rotates from flexion to extension as the wrist is moved from radial to ulnar deviation. In cases of palmar midcarpal instability (PMCI), the proximal row maintains a volar flexed position that will suddenly snap (catch-up clunk) into extension as final extreme ulnar deviation is achieved. Based on cadaveric studies, it is believed that PMCI is caused by laxity of both the dorsal radiotriquetral and palmar ulnar arcuate ligaments, which allows the capitate and hamate to sag within the midcarpal joint.[9] Pain is caused by the abnormal joint reactive forces between the proximal and distal carpal rows secondary to the volar translation of the proximal row in conjunction with a volar intercalated segmental instability (VISI) pattern.[9] A capitolunate instability pattern is seen with laxity present within the radiolunate ligaments and the extrinsic stabilizers of the scaphoid.[9]

The scaphoid and lunate are connected via the palmar and dorsal collagen fascicles of the SL ligament and a proximal region composed of fibrocartilage.[13] The dorsal SL ligaments are thicker and are the main stabilizers of the SL joint[19] while the SL interosseous ligament allows for rotation of the scaphoid on the lunate.[20]

The DRUJ is composed of the pronator quadratus, extensor carpi ulnaris, interosseous membrane (IOM), DRUJ capsule, the triangular fibrocartilage (TFC) articular disk, and the palmar and dorsal radioulnar ligaments.[21] Isolated rupture of the deep fibers of the TFC (palmar and dorsal ligamentum subcruentum) can cause DRUJ instability.[22] Only 25% of the peripheral segments of the TFC articular disk are vascularized, and, therefore, repairs of central disk tears do not heal well.[23]

Imaging

When examining the wrist for ligament injuries, it is also important to obtain standard radiographs to identify acute osseous abnormalities and deformities caused by chronic injuries. Obtaining quality radiographs is important, as the assessment of a joint on a rotated radiograph or with too few views may lead to a missed injury.

When evaluating wrist pain, a full set of radiographs should include a posteroanterior (PA), lateral, scaphoid (PA in ulnar deviation), and a 45-degree semi-pronated oblique view.

The PA view will allow the examiner to assess Gilula's lines[24] to determine if the normal carpal relationships are intact. The PA radiograph also aids in determining if there is a deformity pattern in the wrist. In dorsal intercalated segmental instability (DISI), the lunate is a triangular wedge shape, whereas it has a moonlike configuration in VISI.[25] On the clenched fist view,[26] voluntary grip imparts an axial compression to the carpus and may accentuate SL dissociation. A carpal tunnel view may also be indicated to assess the ventral aspects of the pisiform, trapezium, and hook of the hamate.[27]

Various radiographic characteristics are associated with disruption of the SL ligament. The Terry Thomas sign[28] is an abnormally increased space between the scaphoid and the lunate compared to the contralateral side, or a SL gap of greater than 5 mm.[29] In cases of a palmar-flexed scaphoid, the AP view may demonstrate a "scaphoid ring" sign in which the scaphoid tuberosity projects in the coronal plane as a radiodense circle over the distal two-thirds of the scaphoid.[6] An increased SL angle, greater than 60 degrees, is often seen on the lateral wrist radiograph and represents a palmarly tilted scaphoid in SL dissociation.[24] Often, by the time significant abnormalities are appreciated on plain radiographs, the injury is considered chronic (ie, out of the window where acute repair can be performed).

Lunotriquetral (LT) ligament injuries are more subtle, with 2 signs seen on plain radiographs. A step off on the PA radiograph between the lunate and triquetrum can indicate an intercarpal injury; and a VISI deformity, with the lunate flexed, on the lateral radiograph can indicate an LT injury. Magnetic resonance imaging (MRI) can provide a direct visualization of the carpal ligaments. The sensitivity and specificity of MRI in SL tear is between 59% and 77% and 70% and 83%, respectively. In LT tears, the sensitivity of MRI is 30% to 50%, and the specificity is 4% to 97%.[30]

When evaluating for DRUJ instability, a true lateral scaphopisocapitate view should be obtained. A rotated lateral radiograph can suggest DRUJ malalignment, but the examiner should carefully evaluate the view. In a true lateral radiograph, the palmar cortex of the pisiform overlies the central third of the interval between the palmar cortices of the distal scaphoid pole and the capitate head.[31] A "cross-table," lateral stress view with the patient holding a 5-lb weight and the forearm in pronation can exacerbate DRUJ instability.[32] Ulnar variance, the difference in length between the radius and ulna, can be measured by the distance between a line through the distal ulnar aspect of the radius perpendicular to its longitudinal axis and the distal cortical rim of the ulnar head.[33]

Treatment

Throughout the management of perilunate dislocations, median nerve function should be followed closely as a progressive median nerve deficit is an indication for urgent carpal tunnel release.[34] A closed reduction in the emergency department should be done urgently with the initial placement of finger traps and 10 lbs of traction for 10 minutes. As traction and counter pressure on the volar surface of the lunate are maintained, the wrist is initially placed into dorsiflexion followed by volar flexion to allow the head of the capitate to slip back into the sulcus of the lunate.[35] Surgery can be delayed up to 1 week to allow for decreased swelling if the dislocation can be maintained through closed reduction.[35] Controversy exists as to whether perilunate dislocations should be treated with a dorsal only or a combined dorsal and volar approach. Those who advocate the dorsal approach generally combine it with a carpal tunnel release but do not formally repair the volar ligaments, with the dorsal incision allowing exposure of the dorsal SL ligament for repair and anatomic reduction and fixation of the scaphoid.[34] Others believe that the volar ulnar approach is necessary to repair the disrupted volar capsule and decompress the median nerve in the carpal tunnel and the ulnar nerve in Guyon's canal.[34] Fractures are reduced with the use of Kirschner wires and headless compression screws followed by the restoration of the SL angle to avoid a DISI deformity.[34] Patients are initially placed in a postoperative splint and then converted at 2 weeks to a cast for 8 to 10 weeks.

Symptomatic partial SL ruptures can be treated with arthroscopic débridement of the unstable remnants and reduction and percutaneous pinning of the SL joint with Kirschner wires for 8 weeks.[36] Complete tears of the SL ligament, when diagnosed acutely (up to 6 weeks), should be treated with an open ligament repair and K-wire pinning, with some authors advocating a dorsal capsulodesis.[37] In more chronic presentations, options for treatment of complete SL tears include the Blatt capsulodesis, with a strip of dorsal capsule anchored to the distal scaphoid to act as a tether to prevent hyperflexion and instability[38]; a soft-tissue reconstruction using a strip of the dorsal intercarpal ligament inserted with suture anchors into both the scaphoid and the lunate[39]; or a modified Brunelli tendon reconstruction with a slip of the flexor carpi radialis (FCR) tendon passed through the distal pole of the scaphoid from volar to dorsal with the FCR then anchored to the lunate.[40] If midcarpal or radioscaphoid arthritis is already present, salvage options for SL advanced collapse include proximal row carpectomy, scaphoid excision and "four corner" fusion, or total wrist arthrodesis, depending on the amount and location of the cartilage loss.[41,42]

Acute LT injuries without a VISI deformity or dissociation should initially be treated with cast immobilization with careful molding and a pad underneath the pisiform to maintain optimal alignment.[43] If a dissociation or deformity is present, or after nonoperative management fails, the LT interosseous ligament can be directly repaired to the site of avulsion or reconstructed with a tendon graft. Reconstruction avoids the loss of motion that is associated with LT arthrodesis.[43] In cases of midcarpal or radiocarpal arthritis or positive ulnar variance, an ulnar shortening procedure may be performed.

Palmar midcarpal instability is initially treated nonoperatively with nonsteroidal anti-inflammatory medications, activity modification, and splinting. In mild cases, it may be treated with reefing of the dorsal radiotriquetral ligament.[9] More advanced cases of PMCI can be treated with a limited midcarpal arthrodesis.[44]

Capitolunate instability can be stabilized by suturing the volar radioscaphocapitate to the long radiolunate ligament on the radial side and tethering the capitotriquetral and ulnotriquetral ligaments on the ulnar side.[9] In patients with radial midcarpal instability associated with periscaphoid ligamentous laxity, scaphotrapeziotrapezoid fusion may be an option.[45]

The Hand

History

Injuries to the hand ligaments most commonly occur at the proximal interphalangeal (PIP) joints and at the metacarpophalangeal (MCP) joints, with MCP joint injuries primarily noted in the thumb. In PIP dislocations, patients typically report an axial compression injury with their digit in hyperextension.

Other injuries to the PIP joint include the volar plate injury occurring after a "jamming" trauma to the digit.

Injuries to the thumb MCP joint commonly result in an ulnar collateral ligament (UCL) injury in basketball players or skiers after a fall or other direct trauma, forcing their outstretched hand into an exaggerated position with the thumb in the abducted position.[46] In contrast, the less common radial collateral ligament (RCL) injury of the thumb MCP joint is caused by a hyperextension injury, which may be combined with adduction.[47] In the other digits, the RCL stabilizing the finger MCP joint is injured after forced ulnar deviation with the MCP in flexion[48] and is far more common than UCL injury.[49]

Examination

In cases of PIP dislocation, the patient generally presents in significant pain with an obvious deformity of the digit. It is helpful to examine the finger under digital or wrist block anesthesia, as this also provides pain relief for treatment.[50] The patient should be assessed for active stability, his or her ability to move the digit through the full normal range of motion, and passive stability, with the examiner applying a gentle lateral stress at the joint in full extension and various degrees of flexion. Identifying the degree of flexion when redisplacement occurs allows the surgeon to determine the best position for joint immobilization during splinting.

Patients presenting with an isolated MCP collateral ligament rupture outside the thumb will report tenderness at the RCL or UCL insertion on the radial volar base of the proximal phalanx. Pain and instability will be elicited by ulnar or radial deviation of this digit in full flexion (90 degrees) at the MCP joint.

Patients with acute UCL injuries of the thumb MCP joint present with tenderness, pain, and swelling along the ulnar border of the joint.[46] The thumb should be stressed in both extension and 40 degrees of flexion and compared with the contralateral side. Thirty to 35 degrees of laxity on the ulnar side or 15 degrees more motion with stress than the contralateral side are usually diagnostic of a complete tear. When the force of the injury causes the torn proximal collateral ligament to lie superficial and proximal to the adductor aponeurosis, the Stener lesion,[51] a fullness or mass, will be palpable at the proximal ulnar edge of the MCP joint. In contrast, a partially torn UCL will demonstrate laxity but will have a discrete endpoint.

In tears of the thumb RCL, patients present with diffuse MCP joint swelling and pain with strenuous use of the thumb, such as opening a large jar lid or a doorknob.[47] Partial injuries have a clear endpoint when the MCP joint is stressed, as opposed to a complete RCL rupture in which there may be 15 degrees or more of increased laxity compared to the contralateral thumb, or 30 degrees of laxity in full extension.[52]

Pathoanatomy

Thick collateral ligaments comprising the lateral joint capsule of the PIP joint serve as the primary restraints to radial and ulnar deviation of the joint.[53] The volar plate, which forms the floor of the PIP joint, becomes the primary stabilizer to lateral deviation when the collateral ligaments are incompetent or torn.[53] Collateral ligament injuries are divided into 3 grades. Grade I is a sprain in which the ligament is in continuity but has fiber disruption and no gross instability; Grade II is macroscopically intact with microscopic tearing and laxity; and Grade III is a complete tear of the ligament with gross instability. The majority of collateral ligament failures tend to occur at their proximal end.[53] Dorsal PIP dislocations are also categorized into 3 types. Type I represents partial or complete avulsion of the volar plate with a minor disruption to the collateral ligaments (the volar plate injury); Type II has a major split in the ligaments; and Type III is a fracture dislocation whose stability is defined by the percentage of disruption of the volar articular segment.

The majority of thumb MCP joint injuries occur at the distal insertion of the UCL.[54] In complete tears, the adductor aponeurosis can become interposed between the avulsed ligament and its insertion on the base of the proximal phalanx, known as a Stener lesion.[51] In contrast, the abductor aponeurosis has a broad insertion on the proximal phalanx, and therefore RCL injuries have no associated interposition lesion.

Imaging

Injuries to the PIP joint should be evaluated with plain radiographs, which include a true lateral of the PIP joint. Small volar fractures of the base of the middle phalanx represent volar plate injuries, while fracture dislocations of the

PIP joint must be carefully evaluated for the size of the articular fracture fragments. Pure dislocations must be evaluated for direction of dislocation, with dorsal displacement of the middle phalanx the most common pattern.

In suspected isolated RCL ruptures of the MCP joint, a Brewerton view should be obtained to look for avulsed bony fragments.[55] For thumb collateral ligament injuries, the radiographs should be obtained prior to stressing the joint. A lateral radiograph may show a volar subluxation in a thumb RCL injury whereas the anteroposterior (AP) radiograph may reveal an avulsion fracture or ulnar deviation of the proximal phalanx on the metacarpal. For UCL injuries, ultrasound imaging has been shown to have a sensitivity of 88% and a specificity of 83% for identifying Stener lesions.[56]

Treatment

The key to treating PIP joint injuries is educating the patient that swelling and stiffness may persist for up to 6 months. Type I dorsal PIP injuries, consistent with volar plate injuries, can be treated with immobilization of the joint for 7 days for soft-tissue recovery. Complete dislocations (Type II injuries) should be splinted in up to 30 degrees of flexion at the PIP joint for 1 week to 10 days, while allowing full flexion into the palm, before beginning active exercises with the finger buddy-taped to the adjacent digit. Stable Type III dislocations, with disruption of less than 30% of the volar articular surface, can be treated with 3 weeks of dorsal block splinting.[57] Extension block splinting requires weekly x-rays and may not be successful in larger fragments or in patients with short or swollen fingers.

Unstable PIP joint injuries require fixation of the fracture fragments through dynamic skeletal traction, open reduction and internal fixation (ORIF), or volar plate arthroplasty. Although dynamic traction has been shown to have up to 86 degrees of flexion at 2 years, there is a high rate of pin tract complications, it is uncomfortable for the patient, and it may not fully restore the articular surface.[58] ORIF allows for early range of motion and directly restores the articular surface with use of Kirschner wires or lag screws.[59] In volar plate arthroplasty, the volar plate is advanced into the middle phalanx, and the PIP joint is typically stabilized with K-wires in 20 to 30 degrees of flexion for 3 weeks before starting range of motion.[60] Complications of this procedure include redisplacement, angulation, flexion contractures, and dorsal interphalangeal joint (DIPJ) stiffness. The hemi-hamate resurfacing arthroplasty is a newer described treatment in which a portion of articular distal hamate is used to resurface the comminuted, impacted surface of the base of the middle phalanx.[61]

Stable isolated RCL or UCL tears of the finger MCP joints are treated nonoperatively with immobilization in 30 degrees of flexion for 3 weeks.[48] If the joint remains stable with ulnar stress after 3 weeks, the patient can be progressed to gentle range-of-motion exercises with the finger buddy-taped to the adjacent digit for 3 weeks. If on initial presentation the patient has a grossly unstable joint, a large displaced avulsion fragment off the base of the proximal phalanx, or has subsequently failed nonoperative management, a surgical reconstruction using bone anchors or mini-screws to repair the ligament or bony fragment, which is generally avulsed from the base of the proximal phalanx, should be performed.

Acute partial ruptures of the thumb UCL can be treated with 4 weeks in a thumb spica short arm cast, followed by active and passive range of motion with or without a protective splint.[46] Strenuous activity involving the thumb should be avoided for 3 months. For complete tears, or those associated with a large avulsion fracture at the ulnar base of the proximal phalanx, 2 mm or more of displacement, or articular incongruity, surgical intervention is recommended. The ligament can be reattached at its bony insertion using pullout sutures or bone anchors and immobilized for approximately 4 weeks.[46]

Partial tears of the thumb RCL should be treated nonoperatively following the same protocol as partial UCL injuries. A complete tear can be treated with surgery to include an abductor advancement, either alone or in combination with a repair and/or reefing of the RCL remnant.[62]

CONCLUSION

The early identification and correct diagnosis of wrist and hand ligament injuries is important in treating these injuries acutely. Through the use of a focused history and physical exam, the pathology can be determined with only basic radiographs to confirm the diagnosis (Table 8-3). The

Table 8-3

Helpful Hints

CONDITIONS	COMPLAINTS	EXAMINATION FINDINGS	IMAGING STUDIES
Scapholunate dissociation	Weakness in grip, dorsal pain over SL interval	Positive Watson's scaphoid shift test, positive scapholunate ballottement test	Clenched fist radiograph, Terry Thomas sign on AP view
Triangular fibro-cartilage complex tear	Tenderness to palpation in the soft depression between the pisiform and ulnar styloid	Positive ulnocarpal stress test	
Distal radioulnar joint injury	Ulnar-sided wrist pain	Positive take press and piano key tests	Lateral scaphopisocapitate view
Proximal interphalangeal joint dislocation	Pain and obvious deformity of the digit	Degree of flexion when redisplacement occurs	True lateral radiograph of the PIPJ
Thumb metacarpophalangeal joint ulnar collateral ligament injury	Tenderness, pain, and swelling along ulnar border of joint	Thirty to 35 degrees of laxity on the ulnar side, or 15 degrees greater motion with stress than the contralateral side	Ultrasound to identify Stener lesion
Thumb metacarpophalangeal joint radial collateral ligament injury	Diffuse MCP joint swelling and pain, pain with opening a jar	Fifteen degrees or more of increased laxity compared to the contralateral thumb, or 30 degrees of laxity in full extension	Brewerton view

contralateral wrist and hand should always be used as the comparison for what is normal in each patient. With acute treatment, chronic pain and deformity of the wrist and hand can be avoided.

REFERENCES

1.   Garcia-Elias M, Dobyns JH, Cooney WP, Linscheid RL. Traumatic axial dislocations of the carpus. *J Hand Surg.* 1989;14A:446-457.
2.   Mayfield JK. Mechanism of carpal injuries. *Clin Orthop.* 1980;149:45-54.
3.   Leslie IJ. Carpal instability. *Curr Orthop.* 1994;8:14-22.
4.   Duncan KH, Lewis RC. Scapholunate instability following ganglion cyst excision. *Clin Orthop Rel Res.* 1988;228:250-253.
5.   Crawford GP, Taleisnik J. Rotatory subluxation of the scaphoid after excision of dorsal carpal ganglion and wrist manipulation—A case report. *J Hand Surg.* 1983;8:921-925.
6.   Ruby LK. Carpal instability. *J Bone Joint Surg.* 1995;77A:476-487.
7.   Pin PG, Young VL, Gilula LA, Weeks PM. Management of chronic lunotriquetral ligament tears. *J Hand Surg.* 1989;14A:77-83.
8.   Christodoulou I, Bainbridge LC. Clinical diagnosis of triquetrolunate ligament injuries. *J Hand Surg.* 1999;24B:598-600.
9.   Lichtman DM, Wroten ES. Understanding midcarpal instability. *J Hand Surg.* 2006;31A:491-498.
10. Morrissy RT, Nalebuff EA. Dislocation of the distal radioulnar joint: Anatomy and clues to prompt diagnosis. *Clin Orthop Rel Res.* 1979;144:154-158.
11. Geissler WB, Freeland AE. Arthroscopically assisted reduction of intraarticular distal radial fractures. *Clin Orthop Rel Res.* 1996;327:125-134.
12. Chidgey LK. Chronic wrist pain. *Orthop Clin N Am.* 1992;23:49-64.
13. Watson HK, Ashmead D, Makhlouf MV. Examination of the scaphoid. *J Hand Surg.* 1988;13A:657-660.
14. Lichtman DM, Schneider JR, Swafford AR, Mack GR. Ulnar midcarpal instability—clinical and laboratory analysis. *J Hand Surg.* 1981;6A:515-523.
15. Tay SC, Tomita K, Berger RA. The "Ulnar Fovea Sign" for defining ulnar wrist pain: An analysis of sensitivity and specificity. *J Hand Surg.* 2007;32A:438-444.
16. Forman TA, Forman SK, Rose NE. A clinical approach to diagnosing wrist pain. *Am Fam Phys.* 2005;72:1753-1758.
17. Nakamura R, Horii E, Imaeda T, Nakao E, Kato H, Watanabe K. The ulnocarpal stress test in the diagnosis of ulnar-sided wrist pain. *J Hand Surg.* 1997;22B:719-723.
18. Mason WTM, Hargreaves DG. Arthroscopic thermal capsulorrhaphy for palmar midcarpal instability. *J Hand Surg.* 2007;32B:411-416.
19. Sokolow C, Saffar P. Anatomy and histology of the scapholunate ligament. *Hand Clin.* 2001;17:77-81.

20. Kauer JMG. The mechanism of the carpal joint. *Clin Orthop Rel Res.* 1986;202:16-26.
21. Chidgey LK, Dell PC, Bittar ES, Spanier SS. Histologic anatomy of the triangular fibrocartilage. *J Hand Surg.* 1991;16A:1084-1100.
22. Kleinman WB. Stability of the distal radioulna joint: Biomechanics, pathophysiology, physical diagnosis, and restoration of function. What we have learned in 25 years. *J Hand Surg.* 2007;32A:1086-1106.
23. Mikic Z. The blood supply of the human distal radioulnar joint and the microvasculature of its articular disk. *Clin Orthop Rel Res.* 1992;275:19-28.
24. Gilula LA, Weeks PM. Post-traumatic ligamentous instabilities of the wrist. *Radiology.* 1978;129:641-651.
25. Cantor RM, Braunstein EM. Diagnosis of dorsal and palmar rotation of the lunate on a frontal radiograph. *J Hand Surg.* 1988;13A:187-193.
26. Metz VM, Gilula LA. Is this scapholunate joint and its ligament abnormal? *J Hand Surg.* 1993;18A:746-755.
27. Gilula LA, Destouet JM, Weeks PM, Young LV, Wray RC. Roentgenographic diagnosis of the painful wrist. *Clin Orthop Rel Res.* 1984;187:52-64.
28. Frankel VH. The Terry-Thomas sign. *Clin Orthop Rel Res.* 1977;129:321-322.
29. Cautilli GP, Wehbe MA. Scapho-lunate distance and cortical ring sign. *J Hand Surg.* 1991;16A:501-503.
30. Moser T, Dosch JC, Moussaoui A, Dietemann JL. Wrist ligament tears: Evaluation of MRI and combined MDCT and MR arthrography. *Am J Roentgenol.* 2007;188:278-1286.
31. Yang Z, Mann FA, Gilula LA, Haerr C, Larsen CF. Scaphopisocapitate alignment: Criterion to establish a neutral lateral view of the wrist. *Radiology.* 1997;205:865-869.
32. Scheker LR, Belliappa PP, Acosta R, German DS. Reconstruction of the dorsal ligament of the triangular fibrocartilage complex. *J Hand Surg.* 1994;19B:310-318.
33. Steyers CM, Blair WF. Measuring ulnar variance: a comparison of techniques. *J Hand Surg.* 1989;14A:607-612.
34. Sauder DJ, Athwal GS, Faber KJ, Roth JH. Perilunate injuries. *Orthop Clin N Am.* 2007;38:279-288.
35. DioGiovanni B, Shaffer J. Treatment of perilunate and transscaphoid perilunate dislocations of the wrist. *Am J Orthop.* 1995;24:818-826.
36. Geissler WB, Freeland AE, Weiss APC, Chow JCY. Techniques of wrist arthroscopy. *J Bone Joint Surg.* 1999;81A:1184-1197.
37. Lavernia CJ, Cohen MS, Taleisnik J. Treatment of scapholunate dissociation by ligamentous repair and capsulodesis. *J Hand Surg.* 1992;17A:354-359.
38. Blatt G. Capsulodesis in reconstructive hand surgery: Dorsal capsulodesis for the unstable scaphoid and volar capsulodesis following excision of the distal ulna. *Hand Clin.* 1987;3:81-102.
39. Viegas SF, Yamaguchi S, Boyd NL, Patterson RM. The dorsal ligaments of the wrist: Anatomy, mechanical properties, and function. *J Hand Surg.* 1999;24A:456-468.

40. Van Den Abbeele KLS, Loh YC, Stanley JK, Trail IA. Early results of a modified Brunelli procedure for scapholunate instability. *J Hand Surg.* 1998;23B:258-261.

41. Tomaino MM, Miller RJ, Cole I, Burton RI. Scapholunate advanced collapse wrist: Proximal row carpectomy or limited wrist arthrodesis with scaphoid excision? *J Hand Surg.* 1994;19A:134-142.

42. Sauerbier M, Trankle M, Linsner G, Bickert B, Germann G. Midcarpal arthrodesis with complete scaphoid excision and interposition bone graft in the treatment of advanced carpal collapse (SNAC/SLAC Wrist): Operative technique and outcome assessment. *J Hand Surg.* 2000;25B:341-345.

43. Shin AY, Battaglia MJ, Bishop AT. Lunotriquetral instability: diagnosis and treatment. *J Am Acad Orthop Surg.* 2000;8:170-179.

44. Lichtman DM, Bruckner JD, Culp RW, Alexander CE. Palmar midcarpal instability: Results of surgical reconstruction. *J Hand Surg.* 1993;18A:307-315.

45. Johnson RP, Carrera GF. Chronic capitolunate instability. *J Bone Joint Surg.* 1986;68A:1164-1176.

46. Heyman P. Injuries to the ulnar collateral ligament of the thumb metacarpophalangeal joint. *J Am Acad Orthop Surg.* 1997;5:224-229.

47. Camp RA, Weatherwax RJ, Miller EB. Chronic posttraumatic radial instability of the thumb metacarpophalangeal joint. *J Hand Surg.* 1980;5A:221-225.

48. Schubiner JM, Mass DP. Operation for collateral ligament ruptures of the metacarpophalangeal joints of the fingers. *J Bone Joint Surg.* 1989;71B:388-389.

49. Aguila MB, Carne JS, Lluch AH. Rupture of the ulnar collateral ligament of the metacarpophalangeal joint of the index finger. *J Hand Surg.* 2000;25B:108-109.

50. Eaton RG, Littler JW. Joint injuries and their sequelae. *Clin Plast Surg.* 1976;3:85-98.

51. Stener B. Displacement of the ruptured ulnarcollateral ligament of the metacarpophalangeal joint of the thumb. A clinical and anatomical study. *J Bone Joint Surg.* 1962;44B:869-879.

52. Edelstein DM, Kardashian G, Lee SK. Radial collateral ligament injuries of the thumb. *J Hand Surg Am.* 2008;33(5):760-770.

53. Kiefhaber TR, Stern PJ, Grood ES. Lateral stability of the proximal interphalangeal joint. *J Hand Surg.* 1986;11A:661-669.

54. Bowers WH, Hurst LC. Gamekeeper's thumb. Evaluation by arthrography and stress roentgenography. *J Bone Joint Surg.* 1977;59A:519-524.

55. Lane CS. Detecting occult fractures of the metacarpal head: the Brewerton view. *J Hand Surg.* 1977;2:131-133.

56. Kohut G, O'Callaghan B. Gamekeeper's thumb: Ligament localisation by echography. *Ann Chir Main Memb Super.* 1993;12:257-262.

57. Mcelfresh EC, Dobyns JH, O'Brien ET. Management of fracture-dislocation of the proximal interphalangeal joints by extension-block splinting. *J Bone Joint Surg.* 1972;54A:1705-1711.

58. Bain GI, Mehta JA, Heptinstall R, Bria M. Dynamic external fixation for injuries of the proximal interphalangeal joint. *J Hand Surg.* 1998;80B:1014-1019.

59. Green A, Smith J, Redding M, Akelman E. Acute open reduction and rigid internal fixation of proximal interphalangeal joint fracture dislocation. *J Hand Surg.* 1992;17A:512-517.
60. Durham-Smith G, McCarten GM. Volar plate arthroplasty for closed proximal interphalangeal joint injuries. *J Hand Surg.* 1992;17B:422-428.
61. Calfee RP, Kiefhaber TR, Sommerkamp TG, Stern PJ. Hemi-hamate arthroplasty provides functional reconstruction of acute and chronic proximal interphalangeal fracture-dislocations. *J Hand Surg.* 2009;34A:1232-1241.
62. Durham JW, Khuri S, Kim MH. Acute and late radial collateral ligament injuries of the thumb metacarpophalangeal joint. *J Hand Surg.* 1993;18A:232-237.

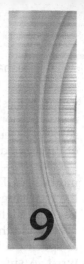

9

NEUROPATHY

Jason M. Erpelding, MD and Anthony J. Lauder, MD

INTRODUCTION

Compression neuropathy of the upper extremity is a chronic condition whereby a peripheral nerve is subjected to constrictive or tensile forces that impair the normal physiological processes of the nerve. This condition contrasts with acute neuropathy, which most frequently occurs from rapid compression in the traumatic setting. Normal and variant anatomical sources of compression come in many forms, including fibrous or fibro-osseous tunnels, traversing myotendinous structures, vascular leashes, post-traumatic deformity, and nerve subluxation. A thorough understanding of these anatomic relationships is essential for the accurate diagnosis and management of these conditions.

Compressive neuropathies are a common source of patient morbidity. The prevalence appears to be increasing, most likely arising from increased awareness, better testing modalities, and higher rates of obesity. The median, radial, and ulnar nerves and their respective branches are subject to dysfunction at specific anatomic locations about the elbow, forearm, and wrist. A single nerve compressed at varying points along its course produces the characteristic clinical findings of sensory and/or motor dysfunction seen in the various compression neuropathies. Sensory dysfunction can range from tingling to dense anesthesia, while motor symptoms can vary from weakness to frank paralysis (Table 9-1). The most common compressive neuropathy of the upper extremity is carpal tunnel syndrome, affecting 1% or more of the general population.[1] Cubital tunnel, or compression of the ulnar nerve at the elbow, is the second most common compression neuropathy of the upper extremity. The socioeconomic impact of these conditions can be staggering, with estimated annual costs for carpal tunnel syndrome exceeding $2 billion in the United States.[1,2]

In addition to anatomic factors, multiple systemic and occupational factors have been associated with the development of compression neuropathies including diabetes, obesity, pregnancy, rheumatoid arthritis, thyroid disorders, renal disease, alcoholism, and the use of heavy vibratory machinery.[1,3] The recognition of these potential contributing and aggravating factors along with an accurate, timely diagnosis and treatment are key to obtaining the best possible outcomes.

HISTORY

Obtaining a very thorough history and physical exam is essential for accurately diagnosing the site or sites of nerve involvement in compressive neuropathies. The onset, duration, progression of symptoms, and history of antecedent trauma should be explored. A history of sensory changes with respect to known dermatomal distributions, weakness of muscle groups with a common innervation, and areas of localizable

Table 9-1

Helpful Hints

NERVE COMPRESSION SITE	SIGNS/SYMPTOMS	SYNDROME
Median		
Wrist	Thumb, index, middle, ring finger numbness and tingling (often nocturnal)	Carpal tunnel syndrome
	Thenar ache/atrophy	
Forearm	Thumb, index, middle, ring finger numbness and tingling (nocturnal symptoms absent)	Pronator syndrome
	Pinch weakness	
	Exacerbation with pronation/elbow flexion	
	No sensory deficits	Anterior interosseous nerve syndrome
Ulnar		
Wrist	Ring and small finger numbness (dorsal hand sparing) Variable intrinsic weakness, finger coordination loss	Ulnar tunnel syndrome
Elbow	Ring, small finger, dorsal hand numbness	Cubital tunnel syndrome
	Clumsiness, intrinsic weakness, dropping objects	
Radial		
Elbow	Minimal to no sensory changes	Posterior interosseous nerve syndrome
	Thumb and finger extensor weakness	
	Lateral elbow/dorsal forearm ache	Radial tunnel syndrome
	No sensory or motor deficits	
	Pain, numbness, burning of dorsoradial wrist to dorsal thumb and index fingers	Wartenberg's syndrome

pain will help direct the practitioner to a differential diagnosis. Furthermore, a thorough occupational history should be evaluated. Significant controversy exists regarding compression neuropathy and its relationship to work-related activities. While some occupations—including meat butchering and use of vibratory tools—seem to be risk factors for developing carpal tunnel syndrome, most other occupations have not been directly linked to the development of compression neuropathy. Careful note of the patient's overall health and other medical conditions can also be very helpful for ruling out issues that can result in nerve symptoms and dysfunction. For instance, patients with uncontrolled diabetes will often have vague complaints of bilateral upper extremity numbness and pain, which can be confused with carpal tunnel syndrome. Unfortunately, patients with diabetic neuropathy will not benefit from the treatment regimen normally implemented for carpal tunnel syndrome.

Symptoms of compression neuropathy are typically slow to progress and present for 6 months or more prior to presentation. One must be cognizant of other syndromes, which can mimic peripheral nerve compression neuropathy, as their treatment differs significantly. Parsonage-Turner syndrome is a self-resolving brachial neuritis that typically follows a viral illness or immunization.[4,5] Patients often present with transient shoulder pain, upper extremity weakness, paresthesias, and anterior interosseous nerve (AIN) palsy. Thoracic outlet syndrome, or compression of the brachial plexus, can imitate more distal ulnar nerve compressive neuropathies. However, in thoracic outlet syndrome, most symptoms can be reproduced with overhead activities. Finally, one should be aware that nerves can be compressed at multiple levels. One example of this has been termed the *double crush* phenomenon, in which cervical radiculopathy is superimposed on a peripheral compression neuropathy.[1] Most commonly, this occurs with C5-6 radiculopathy and carpal tunnel syndrome.

Several neuropathies are associated with compression of the median nerve, including carpal tunnel syndrome, pronator syndrome, and anterior interosseous syndrome. Carpal tunnel syndrome, or compression of the median nerve at the wrist, can lead to nocturnal symptoms; weakness; a history of dropping objects; and numbness and tingling of the thumb, index, and middle fingers. Patients may also complain of thenar

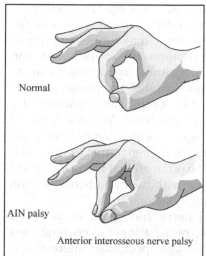

Normal

AIN palsy

Anterior interosseous nerve palsy

Figure 9-1. An anterior interosseous nerve palsy leads to a loss of precision pinch due to weakness of the flexor pollicis longus and flexor digitorum profundus to the index finger. AIN, anterior interosseous nerve.

eminence aching, with atrophy in severe cases. Complaints of bilateral symptoms are present in 60% of cases.[6] More proximal compression of the median nerve in the forearm can lead to pronator syndrome and complaints of pain and paresthesias in the thumb, index, and middle fingers. Unlike carpal tunnel syndrome, patients with pronator syndrome will often not have nocturnal symptoms, but rather a history of exacerbations related to strenuous activities requiring repetitive forearm pronation with an extended elbow.[7] Anterior interosseous syndrome is a motor palsy with no significant sensory changes. Patients predominantly complain of difficulty with pinch activities stemming from weakness in the flexor pollicis longus (FPL) and flexor digitorum profundus (FDP) to the index finger (Figure 9-1). Volar wrist pain may also be present as the terminal branches of the AIN innervate the volar wrist capsule.

Ulnar nerve compression neuropathy is composed of cubital and ulnar tunnel syndromes. Cubital tunnel symptoms include medial elbow pain, paresthesias, and numbness of the small and ring fingers that extend onto the dorsum of the hand. Involvement of the ulnar forearm suggests more proximal compression that occurs with thoracic outlet syndrome. Night-time symptoms are common in patients who sleep with their elbows in a flexed position. Grip weakness may also be present. Clumsiness and intrinsic hand weakness can develop as compression progresses. Ulnar tunnel syndrome, stemming from ulnar nerve compression at the wrist, can occur concomitantly with carpal tunnel syndrome in up to one-third of cases.[8] Unlike cubital tunnel syndrome, patients with ulnar tunnel syndrome will not complain of paresthesias or numbness on the dorsum of the hand. Variable intrinsic muscle weakness or loss of finger coordination may be present. Inquire about trauma to the hypothenar area to rule out a hook of the hamate fracture. The occupational use of handheld heavy equipment or hammering with the hypothenar portion of the hand may be a contributing factor.

Compression of the radial nerve can result in posterior interosseous nerve syndrome, radial tunnel syndrome, and Wartenberg's syndrome. Although posterior interosseous nerve syndrome and radial tunnel syndrome are similar with regard to the location of the compression of the radial nerve around the elbow, they differ significantly in the symptoms caused. Posterior interosseous nerve syndrome results in motor deficits (weakness of finger and thumb extensors) with little to no sensory changes. Patients with radial tunnel syndrome will complain of a deep ache or cramp over the lateral elbow and dorsal forearm very similar to a lateral epicondylitis. Radial tunnel syndrome will not lead to any motor or sensory complaints. Wartenberg's syndrome, or compression of the superficial branch of the radial nerve in the forearm, will lead to pain, numbness, and burning sensations over the dorso-radial aspect of the wrist. Symptoms will often radiate into the dorsum of the thumb and index finger.

EXAMINATION

The physical examination for localization of compression neuropathy should be very thorough so as to identify all possible sites of pathology. It must encompass the entire upper extremity from the cervical spine and brachial plexus to the wrist and hand. Key components of the examination include a general inspection looking for skin and color changes, motor and sensory testing, Tinel's sign testing, and specific provocative maneuvers known to elicit symptoms by increasing pressure on specific nerves (Table 9-2).

Table 9-2

Methods for Examining in Compression Neuropathy

EXAMINATION	TECHNIQUE		SIGNIFICANCE
C-Spine/Thoracic Outlet			
Spurling's maneuver	The Spurling's maneuver is performed with the neck extended and the head turned to the affected side while being axially loaded. It is considered a positive test if radiating symptoms down the affected side are reproduced.	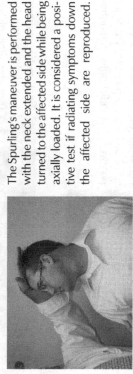	Radiating pain down the affected side can indicate cervical root involvement.
Wright's maneuver	The Wright's maneuver is performed with hyperabduction of the shoulder on the affected side. A positive test occurs when the radial pulse decreases.	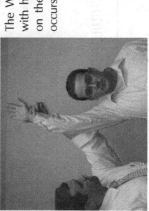	A diminished radial pulse can indicate thoracic outlet syndrome.

(continued)

Methods for Examining in Compression Neuropathy

Table 9-2 (continued)

EXAMINATION	TECHNIQUE		SIGNIFICANCE
Adson's maneuver	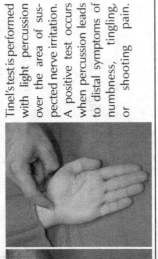	The Adson's maneuver is performed with abduction, extension, and external rotation of the shoulder. The patient is then asked to rotate his or her head toward the affected side while taking a deep breath. The test is positive if the radial pulse diminishes.	A diminished radial pulse can indicate thoracic outlet syndrome.

Nerve (General)

| Tinel's test | 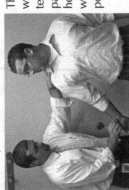 | Tinel's test is performed with light percussion over the area of suspected nerve irritation. A positive test occurs when percussion leads to distal symptoms of numbness, tingling, or shooting pain. | Shooting pain or tingling in the area of nerve distribution can indicate nerve irritation. |

(continued)

Table 9-2 (continued)

Methods for Examining in Compression Neuropathy

EXAMINATION	TECHNIQUE	SIGNIFICANCE
Semmes-Weinstein monofilament test	Semmes and Weinstein described the use of nylon monofilaments of varying thicknesses as a method for assessing cutaneous pressure threshold. Enough pressure should be applied to the monofilament to create a slight "C" shape. Changes in Semmes-Weinstein testing can be the first sign of a compression neuropathy.	Diminished ability to sense monofilaments can be the earliest sign of a compression neuropathy.
Two-point discrimination	Two-point discrimination can also be utilized to assess for compression neuropathy. Enough pressure should be applied to blanch the skin. The test is considered abnormal if the patient's two-point discrimination is 6 mm or greater. 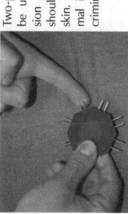	Inability to discriminate 5 mm or less of point separation can be a sign of compression neuropathy.

(continued)

Table 9-2 (continued)

Methods for Examining in Compression Neuropathy

Pronator/ Anterior Interosseous Nerve Syndrome

EXAMINATION	TECHNIQUE	SIGNIFICANCE
Resisted elbow flexion/forearm supinated	With a supinated forearm, the patient is asked to flex the elbow against resistance.	Reproduction of symptoms (numbness/tingling) can indicate compression of the median nerve in the forearm by the lacertus fibrosis or ligament of Struther's.
Resisted forearm pronation/elbow extended	With an extended elbow, the patient is asked to pronate the forearm against resistance.	Reproduction of symptoms (numbness/tingling) can indicate compression of the median nerve in the forearm by the pronator teres.
Resisted proximal interphalangeal (PIP) joint flexion middle finger	Patient is asked to flex the middle finger at the PIP joint against resistance.	Reproduction of symptoms (numbness/tingling) can indicate compression of the median nerve in the forearm by the flexor digitorum superficialis.

(continued)

Table 9-2 (continued)

Methods for Examining in Compression Neuropathy

EXAMINATION	TECHNIQUE	SIGNIFICANCE
Carpal Tunnel Syndrome		
Durkan's compression maneuver	Durkan's compression maneuver is performed by applying pressure over the carpal tunnel (enough to cause skin blanching) for at least 30 seconds. A positive test occurs when the patient's symptoms (numbness/tingling) are reproduced.	Reproduction of symptoms (numbness/tingling) can indicate carpal tunnel syndrome.
Phalen's test	Phalen's test is performed with the patient's wrist flexed against gravity for at least 60 seconds. A test is considered positive when the patient's symptoms (numbness/tingling) are reproduced.	Reproduction of symptoms can indicate carpal tunnel syndrome.

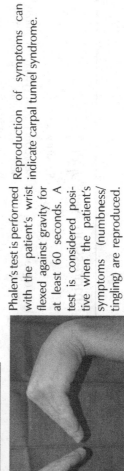

(continued)

Table 9-2 (continued)

Methods for Examining in Compression Neuropathy

EXAMINATION	TECHNIQUE	SIGNIFICANCE
Closed fist test	Patient holds his or her fist clenched tightly for at least 60 seconds.	Reproduction of symptoms (numbness/tingling) can indicate carpal tunnel syndrome.

Cubital Tunnel Syndrome

Froment's sign	A positive Froment's sign occurs with a low ulnar nerve palsy. The patient attempts to compensate for a weak adductor pollicis muscle by flexion at the interphalangeal joint with the flexor pollicis longus. FPL, flexor pollicis longus.	A positive test indicates weakness of the adductor pollicis muscle, which can occur in cubital tunnel syndrome.

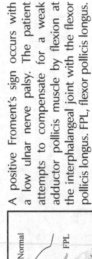

Normal
FPL

Ulnar nerve palsy
FPL

Positive Forment's sign

(continued)

Table 9-2 (continued)

Methods for Examining in Compression Neuropathy

Examination	Technique	Significance
Elbow flexion/forearm supination/wrist extension	Patient is asked to simultaneously flex the elbow, supinate the forearm, and extend the wrist.	Reproduction of symptoms (numbness/tingling) can indicate irritation of the ulnar nerve at the cubital tunnel.
Elbow flexion/compression ulnar nerve at elbow	Patient is asked to flex the elbow while the examiner compresses the ulnar nerve at the elbow.	Reproduction of symptoms (numbness/tingling) can indicate irritation of the ulnar nerve at the cubital tunnel.
Posterior Interosseous Nerve/Radial Tunnel Syndrome		
Point tenderness	Examiner applies firm pressure over the dorsal forearm 5 cm distal to the lateral epicondyle.	Reproduction of symptoms (pain/ache) can indicate compression of the radial nerve and radial tunnel syndrome.
Middle finger test	Patient is asked to simultaneously extend elbow, pronate forearm, and flex wrist while attempting to extend middle and ring fingers against resistance.	Reproduction of symptoms (pain/ache) can indicate compression of the radial nerve and radial tunnel syndrome.
Injection test	One to 2 cc's of lidocaine are injected into the radial tunnel at the point of maximal tenderness.	Relief of patient's symptoms can indicate compression of the radial nerve and radial tunnel syndrome.
Loss finger/thumb extension	Patient asked to actively extend thumb interphalangeal joint and fingers at metacarpophalangeal joints.	Positive test occurs when weakness or paralysis is noted when patient attempts to extend thumb and digits. Test can indicate posterior interosseous nerve (PIN) syndrome.

(continued)

Table 9-2 (continued)

Methods for Examining in Compression Neuropathy

EXAMINATION	TECHNIQUE	SIGNIFICANCE
Wrist extension in radial deviation	Patient is asked to actively extend wrist.	Positive test occurs if wrist extends and radially deviates. This occurs because extensor carpi radialis longus (ECRL) is innervated more proximally than extensor carpi radialis brevis (ECRB). ECRL attaches to base of second metacarpal which leads to radial deviation. Test can indicate PIN syndrome.
Wartenberg's Syndrome Pronation test	Patient is asked to fully pronate forearm.	Reproduction of symptoms (tingling/numbness dorsal hand) can indicate compression of the superficial branch of the radial nerve.

The exam should begin by noting the overall appearance and positioning of the upper extremity. Calluses of the hands, cuts, and abrasions provide evidence for the level of use of the extremity and protective sensation. Post-traumatic deformities must also be evaluated, as they can lead to increased stress on nerves as they traverse the irregularity. The fingers should be partially flexed at rest, and any radial or ulnar-sided clawing should be documented. Abnormal skin color, temperature, or sweat pattern can indicate a disturbance of sympathetic tone. Atrophy of muscle groups with common innervations indicates a chronic process and can be indicative of increased severity.

The cervical spine should be examined next for signs of cervical root involvement. Signs of root involvement are suggested by pain with neck range of motion and a positive Spurling's maneuver (see Table 9-2). Thoracic outlet syndrome can be confirmed if Wright's (see Table 9-2) or Adson's (see Table 9-2) maneuvers are positive.

Following inspection and a cervical spine exam, strength testing is performed to assess for weakness of specific muscle groups innervated by a common peripheral nerve (Table 9-3). A thorough motor exam should also evaluate pinch and grip strength.

The sensory exam should include threshold measurements with Semmes-Weinstein monofilaments (see Table 9-2). Sensory changes identified with this modality are often the first sign of compression neuropathy. As the neuropathy progresses and larger numbers of nerve fibers are affected, deficits in density testing with static and moving two-point discrimination become apparent (see Table 9-2). The sensory exam should follow known nerve-specific dermatomal relationships (Figure 9-2). Another useful technique for localizing sites of nerve compression is a Tinel's test (see Table 9-2). A positive test is elicited when light percussion along the course of the nerve causes tingling or paresthesias in more distal areas supplied by the nerve in question.

Finally, specific tests and provocative maneuvers can be used for particular sites of nerve compression in the upper extremity. Two useful tests for carpal tunnel syndrome include Durkan's compression maneuver and Phalen's test (see Table 9-2). A Durkan's compression maneuver is positive when

Table 9-3

Nerve-Specific Motor Testing

NERVE	LOCATION	MUSCLE GROUP
Median	Wrist	Abductor pollicis brevis, opponens pollicis brevis
	Forearm	Flexor pollicis longus, flexor digitorum profundus to index finger, pronator teres, flexor digitorum superficialis
Ulnar	Wrist	Abductor digiti minimi, first dorsal interosseous
	Elbow	Flexor digitorum profundus of small finger, flexor carpi ulnaris, ulnar intrinsics
Radial	Elbow	Wrist, thumb, and finger extensors

Adapted from Dellon L. Compression neuropathy. In: Trumble TE, Budoff JE, Cornwall R, eds. *Hand, Elbow, & Shoulder: Core Knowledge in Orthopaedics.* Philadelphia, PA: Mosby Elsevier; 2006:234-254.

Figure 9-2. Palmar and dorsal views of the sensory patterns for the median, ulnar, and radial nerves in the hand.

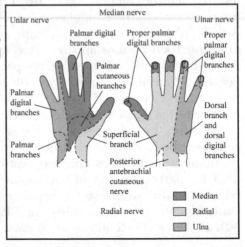

compression of the median nerve at the wrist for 30 to 60 seconds leads to tingling, while Phalen's test is positive if wrist flexion for 60 seconds reproduces symptoms.

Tinel's test can be very useful for diagnosing cubital tunnel syndrome, but 24% of normal subjects have been noted to have a positive test. Cubital tunnel symptoms can also be reproduced with elbow flexion, forearm supination, and wrist extension. However, 10% of normal people will have a positive test.[9,10] Novak and colleagues found that the elbow flexion test combined with direct pressure on the ulnar nerve at the elbow is a more sensitive and specific test.[11] Froment's sign will be positive in severe cases of ulnar nerve compression (see Table 9-2). In contradistinction to those with cubital tunnel syndrome, patients with ulnar tunnel syndrome (ulnar nerve compression at the wrist) will have intact flexor digitorum profundus function to the small finger and normal sensation to the dorsum of the ring and small fingers.[9,12]

Patients with radial tunnel syndrome will have point tenderness over the dorsal forearm about 5 cm distal to the lateral epicondyle, while patients with lateral epicondylitis have pain more directly over the condyle. Asking the patient to extend his or her elbow, pronate his or her forearm, and flex his or her wrist while trying to extend the long and ring fingers against resistance may reproduce painful symptoms in the forearm. Patients with posterior interosseous nerve syndrome will have difficulty or inability to fire the long extensor to the thumb or the common extensors to the metacarpal phalangeal joints of the fingers.[13] The wrist may extend radially in a deviated fashion due to the preserved function of the extensor carpi radialis longus.

PATHOANATOMY

Simply stated, neuropathy develops when compressive pressures exceed those normally tolerated by the nerve in question. The cause of the compression can be of the utmost importance (ie, tumor, post-traumatic deformity, arthritis) but—for the most part—the vast majority of compressive neuropathy stems from idiopathic sources. The histologic changes that occur in the nerve depend on both force and duration of compression.

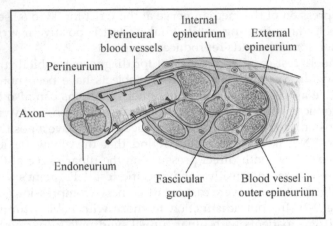

Figure 9-3. Illustration depicting the organization of a peripheral nerve at the microscopic level.

More superficial fibers of the nerve are generally affected first, which explains why the ring and long fingers are normally symptomatic before the index finger and thumb in carpal tunnel syndrome. Furthermore, patient complaints generally correlate with histologic changes, with symptoms becoming more persistent and severe as nerve damage increases.

Whether symptoms and histologic changes result from mechanical factors, ischemic changes, or both remains controversial. Studies have shown that nerve compression of 20 to 30 mm Hg can lead to decreased axonal transport within the nerve as well as decreased venous outflow from the nerve. Intraneural blood flow will be blocked at 60 to 80 mm Hg. Prolonged compression can lead to intraneural edema, nerve demyelination, and ultimately interfascicular fibrosis (Figure 9-3). In the example of carpal tunnel syndrome, Gelberman and colleagues demonstrated mean carpal tunnel pressures of 32 mm Hg in patients with carpal tunnel syndrome and mean carpal tunnel pressures of 2.5 mm Hg in controls.[14] Authors have also shown increased carpal tunnel pressures with wrist flexion, wrist extension, fist formation, and isometric finger flexion against resistance.[14,15]

The double crush phenomenon, first introduced in 1973, is a concept with which the health care provider evaluating for compression neuropathy should be familiar. A nerve that is crushed (compressed) in one location becomes more susceptible to injury at a more distal location. This finding probably stems from proximal compression compromising normal axoplasmic flow, which leads to a tenuousness for nerve well-being downstream. This phenomenon emphasizes the importance of thoroughly evaluating patients with upper extremity compressive neuropathy who are at high risk for concomitant cervical pathology.

General risk factors for compressive neuropathy include obesity, female gender, diabetes, hypothyroidism, rheumatoid arthritis, and excessive alcohol use.

IMAGING/TESTING

Routine radiographs are generally not necessary in classic cases of compression neuropathy. As with everything in medicine, there are always exceptions to this rule. Patients who present with deformity or a prior history of trauma to an area near the site of compression should have x-rays obtained. Radiographs may expose underlying malunions or large osteophytes as the etiology for the patient's neuropathy. In these instances, radiographic information is critical, as surgical decompression of the nerve alone does not address the true cause of the patient's symptoms.

Some patients may present with signs of neuropathy as the initial symptoms of either benign or malignant tumors (Figure 9-4). If tumor is a concern, MRI is an extremely valuable tool for evaluating both the root of the neuropathy as well as the size and extent of the mass. This is especially true with ulnar nerve compression at the wrist (ulnar tunnel syndrome) where benign ganglions are often the source for nerve compression.

Electromyography (EMG) and nerve conduction studies (NCS) are electrodiagnostic studies traditionally used to help diagnose and determine the severity of compressive neuropathy in peripheral nerves. These studies can quantify skeletal muscle dysfunction and evaluate the integrity of motor and sensory nerves.[16] Caution should be exercised when

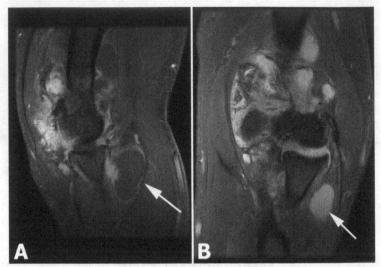

Figure 9-4. (A) Sagital MRI demonstrating a large elbow ganglion (arrow) overlying radial neck. (B) Coronal MRI demonstrating the same ganglion just radial to the radial neck. The mass effect from this ganglion led to a posterior interosseous nerve palsy in this patient.

interpreting results from these tests, however. A meta-analysis in 1993 demonstrated a 33% false-negative rate for EMG/ NCS in patients with carpal tunnel syndrome.[17] Furthermore, Szabo and colleagues demonstrated that carpal tunnel syndrome was correctly diagnosed 86% of the time when the combination of night-time pain, a positive Durkan's compression maneuver, a positive Semmes-Weinstein monofilament test, and a positive Brigham hand diagram were all present. When these 4 findings were absent, the number of patients diagnosed with carpal tunnel syndrome plummeted to 0.68%. Importantly, electrodiagnostic testing did not augment one's ability to diagnose carpal tunnel syndrome in this study.[18]

Although certain limitations make neurodiagnostic studies a poor replacement for a thorough history and physical exam, they are an integral portion of the workup for compression neuropathy.[19] They are particularly useful in ruling out other serious conditions including cervical disk disease, anterior motor neuron disease, central nervous system pathology, and peripheral neuropathy due to systemic illnesses like diabetes mellitus.

Using carpal tunnel syndrome as an example, one can evaluate the abnormal findings expected with neurodiagnostic studies. Nerve conduction studies will reveal decreased amplitude, decreased velocity, and increased latency. In terms of numbers, this translates to a sensory nerve latency greater than 3.5 ms and a motor nerve latency above 4.5 ms. Alterations in the EMG, found in more chronic disease, would include increased insertional activity, fibrillation potentials at rest, and decreased motor unit potential recruitment with muscle contraction.

TREATMENT

Median Nerve Compression: Carpal Tunnel Syndrome

Conservative measures are the mainstay of initial treatment for mild to moderate compression of the median nerve at the wrist. A trial of night-time wrist splinting should be used in any patient without severe disease. Importantly, the splint should keep the wrist in a neutral position. Unfortunately, most off-the-shelf splints will place the wrist in some degree of extension. Fortunately, this can easily be remedied by manually removing the bend built into the splint. Oral medications including nonsteroidal anti-inflammatory drugs and vitamin B6 have some proven effectiveness when combined with night-time wrist splinting. Steroid injections into the carpal tunnel can also be helpful, especially in the patient with an equivocal history and/or exam (Figure 9-5). In these patients, relief from an injection can help make the diagnosis and can be a predictor of significant benefit from surgical release. Finally, some patients will benefit from activity modification to help minimize positions of the hand and/or wrist that place pressure on the median nerve. These modifications may include creating more ergonomic environments at the workplace and/or vocational rehabilitation.

Surgical decompression of the carpal tunnel is indicated in patients who fail conservative measures. Surgical release should also be considered as the initial treatment in patients with signs of severe disease including constant numbness,

Figure 9-5. With a carpal tunnel injection, the needle should be inserted just ulnar to the palmaris longus at a 45-degree angle from proximal to distal. The needle should be advanced in line with the radial aspect of the ring finger. FCR, flexor carpi radialis; FCU, flexor carpi ulnaris.

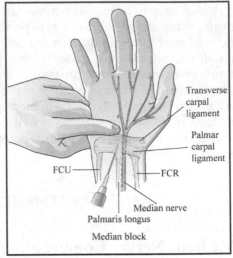

Figure 9-6. The incision for an open carpal tunnel should be along the axis of the radial border of the ring finger and centered over the transverse carpal ligament.

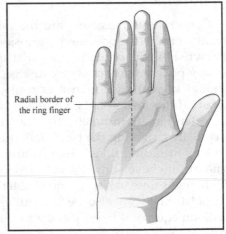

thenar atrophy, or electromyography demonstrating motor denervation. Open, mini-open, and endoscopic releases are available techniques with a common goal of complete transection of the transverse carpal ligament (Figures 9-6 and 9-7). At this time, no particular technique has been shown to be significantly superior. In general, studies comparing open with endoscopic techniques have demonstrated earlier recovery but more frequent major complications with the endoscopic techniques.[20] Importantly, long-term outcomes appear to be

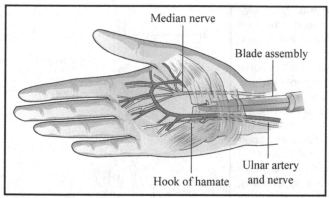

Figure 9-7. An endoscopic release can be performed through a small transverse incision at the distal wrist crease centered over the palmaris longus.

equivalent for any technique implemented. Results are probably most dependent on the decompression method with which the surgeon is most comfortable.

Median Nerve Compression: Pronator Syndrome/Anterior Interosseous Syndrome

Spontaneous dysfunction of the anterior interosseous nerve (paralysis of the flexor pollicis longus and flexor digitorum profundus to the index finger) is most often the result of neuritis. This neuritis has been termed Parsonage-Turner syndrome. The vast majority of patients will have palsy resolution with a watch-and-wait approach. Some have argued that courses of steroids and antivirals can be helpful because this syndrome often follows a viral illness. Although spontaneous recovery has been reported at up to 1 year, some authors have suggested that surgical decompression should be undertaken at 3 months after an EMG has demonstrated no signs of reinnervation.

Pronator syndrome is often successfully treated with observation and activity modification. This is especially true in patients who have a job that requires repetitive flexion and

Figure 9-8. Structures that need to be released or lengthened in the proximal forearm with median nerve compression include the lacertus fibrosis, superficial head of the pronator teres, the flexor digitorum superficialis, and ligament of Struther's. FDS, flexor digitorum superficialis; FDP, flexor digitorum profundus.

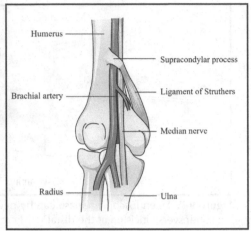

Labels: Humerus, Supracondylar process, Brachial artery, Ligament of Struthers, Median nerve, Radius, Ulna

pronation of the elbow and forearm. Splinting and anti-inflammatory medications can also provide relief for some patients. Symptoms that fail to improve with conservative measures should be treated with surgical intervention. The technique, which is the same for both pronator and anterior interosseous syndromes, involves complete release of the median nerve in the proximal forearm. Structures that need to be released or lengthened include the lacertus fibrosis, superficial head of the pronator teres, the flexor digitorum superficialis fascia, and the ligament of Struthers (if present) (Figures 9-8 and 9-9).

Ulnar Nerve Compression: Ulnar Tunnel Syndrome (Guyon's Canal)

Activity modification, padded gloves, splinting, and anti-inflammatory medications can initially be used to treat ulnar nerve compression at the wrist. An MRI should be obtained prior to implementing treatment to rule out a space-occupying lesion. Space-occupying lesions should be surgically excised. Patients who fail conservative measures should have a surgical decompression through a slightly extended carpal tunnel incision.

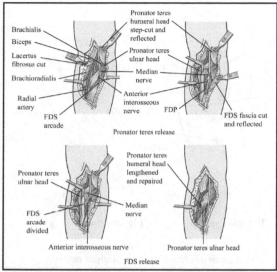

Figure 9-9. In some patients, a ligament of Struther's can be present seen here extending from a humeral supracondylar process to the medial epicondyle.

Ulnar Nerve Compression: Cubital Tunnel Syndrome

Nonoperative treatment is usually successful in patients presenting with mild cubital tunnel. These patients will often benefit from activity modification; specifically, learning to avoid positions that place the ulnar nerve under tension (ie, elbow flexion). Other helpful conservative measures include anti-inflammatory medications, elbow pads, and night-time splints. Night-time splints, which hold the elbow in 30 degrees to 45 degrees of flexion, can be helpful but are often not worn due to discomfort. Surgical intervention is indicated in any patient failing 2 to 4 months of conservative management and in patients who present with severe disease. Surgical techniques include in situ decompression (open and endoscopic), medial epicondylectomy, anterior subcutaneous transposition, and anterior submuscular transposition (Figures 9-10 and 9-11). In a 2008 meta-analysis comparing in situ decompression with anterior transposition procedures, Macadam and colleagues found no statistical differences between the techniques.[21]

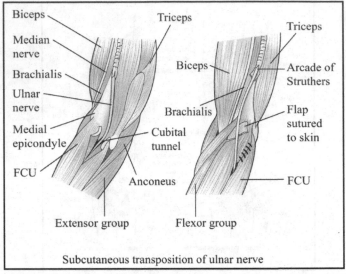

Subcutaneous transposition of ulnar nerve

Figure 9-10. An anterior subcutaneous transposition of the ulnar nerve involves complete decompression, an anterior transposition, and the creation of a fascial sling to prevent a return of the nerve into the cubital tunnel. FCU, flexor carpi ulnaris.

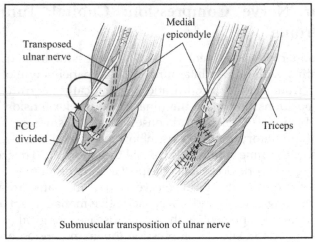

Submuscular transposition of ulnar nerve

Figure 9-11. A submuscular transposition of the ulnar nerve involves complete decompression, an anterior transposition, and creation of muscular tunnel under the flexor/pronator origin. FCU, flexor carpi ulnaris.

There was a slight trend for improved outcomes in the transposition groups.

Radial Nerve Compression: Posterior Interosseous Nerve Syndrome/Radial Tunnel Syndrome

Patients with radial tunnel syndrome have pain similar to lateral epicondylitis without motor symptoms, while patients with posterior interosseous syndrome have weakness of the finger and thumb extensors. However, although the signs and symptoms of the 2 entities are quite different, they are treated in an identical manner. Splinting, activity modification, and anti-inflammatory medications are reasonable initial treatment options. Steroids can be used judiciously by direct injection into the radial tunnel. Not only can an injection relieve symptoms, but it can also help when a specific diagnosis is in question. Surgical intervention can be undertaken in patients who fail the initial conservative measures. At the time of surgery, the radial tunnel must be decompressed with release of the Fibrous bands anterior to the radial head, the Radial recurrent vessels, the fibrous edge of the Extensor carpi radialis brevis, the leading edge of the supinator (Arcade of Frohse), and the distal edge of the Supinator (FREAS) (Figure 9-12).

Radial Nerve Compression—Sensory Radial Nerve Compression (Wartenberg's Syndrome)

Neuropathy of the superficial branch of the radial nerve in the forearm can normally be successfully treated with activity modification, wrist splinting, anti-inflammatory medications, and gentle stretching exercises. Surgery is rarely indicated but, in recalcitrant cases, can be performed with release of the fascia between the brachioradialis and extensor carpi radialis longus.

CONCLUSION

Compression neuropathy is a common cause of morbidity and its etiology can be multifactorial. An accurate diagnosis

Figure 9-12. The radial nerve can be released between the extensor digitorum communis and extensor carpi radialis brevis with the posterior or Thompson approach.

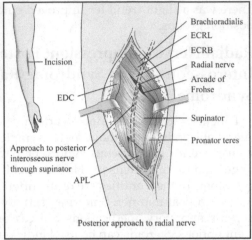

Brachioradialis
ECRL
ECRB
Radial nerve
Arcade of Frohse
Supinator
Pronator teres

Incision

EDC

Approach to posterior interosseous nerve through supinator

APL

Posterior approach to radial nerve

depends on a thorough history and detailed physical exam. Routine radiographs and other imaging modalities are not required but should be liberally used in patients with a history of trauma, deformity, or possible tumor in the area of compression. Treatment begins with conservative measures, which can include activity modification, splinting, anti-inflammatory medications, and judicious use of injections. Surgery should be considered for those who fail conservative management or present with well-established or severe cases. In general, surgical intervention is the same in all cases in that it involves decompression of the nerve at the offending site.

REFERENCES

1. Cranford CS, Ho JY, Kalainov DM, Hartigan BJ. Carpal tunnel syndrome. *J Am Acad Orthop Surg.* 2007;15(9):537-548.
2. Palmer DH, Hanrahan LP. Social and economic costs of carpal tunnel surgery. *Instructional Course Lecture.* 1995;44:167-172.
3. Dellon L. Compression neuropathy. In: Trumble TE, Budoff JE, Cornwall R, eds. Hand, elbow, & shoulder: Core knowledge in orthopaedics. Philadelphia, PA: Mosby Elsevier; 2006:234-254.
4. Tsai P, Steinber DR. Median and radial nerve compression about the elbow. *J Bone Joint Surg Am.* 2008;90(2):420-428.
5. Wong L, Dellon AL. Brachial neuritis presenting as anterior interosseous nerve compression—Implications for diagnosis and treatment: A case report. *J Hand Surg Am.* 1997;22(3):536-539.

6. Trumble TE. Compressive neuropathies. In: Trumble TE, eds. *Principles of hand surgery therapy.* Philadelphia, PA: WB Saunders; 2000:324-342.

7. Lubahn JD, Cermak MB. Uncommon nerve compression syndromes of the upper extremity. *J Am Acad Orthop Surg.* 1998;6(6):378-386.

8. Waugh RP, Pellegrini VD. Ulnar tunnel syndrome. *Hand Clinics.* 2007;23(3):301-310.

9. Elhassan B, Steinmann SP. Entrapment neuropathy of the ulnar nerve. *J Am Acad Orthop Surg.* 2007;15(11):672-681.

10. Rayan GM, Jensen C, Duke J. Elbow flexion test in the normal population. *J Hand Surg Am.* 1992;17(1):86-89.

11. Novak CB, Lee GW, Mackinnon SE, Lay L. Provocative testing for cubital tunnel syndrome. *J Hand Surg Am.* 1994;19(5):817-820.

12. Posner MA. Compressive ulnar neuropathies at the elbow: I. etiology and diagnosis. *J Am Acad Orthop Surg.* 1998;6(5):282-288.

13. Gelberman RH, Eaton R, Urbaniak JR. Peripheral nerve compression. *Instr Course Lect.* 1994;43:31-53.

14. Gelberman RH, Hergenroeder PT, Hargens AR, Lundborg GN, Akeson WH. The carpal tunnel syndrome: A study of carpal pressures. *J Bone Joint Surg Am.* 1981;63(3):380-383.

15. Seradge H, Jia YC, Owens W. In vivo measurement of carpal tunnel pressure in the functioning hand. *J Hand Surg Am.* 1995;20(5):855-859.

16. Strandberg EJ, Mozaffar T, Gupta R. The role of neurodiagnostic studies in nerve injuries and other orthopedic disorders. *J Hand Surg Am.* 2007;32(8):1280-1290.

17. Jablecki CK, Andary MT, So YT, Wilkins DE, Williams FH. Literature review of the usefulness of nerve conduction studies and electromyography for the evaluation of patients with carpal tunnel syndrome. AAEM Quality Assurance Committee. *Muscle Nerve.* 1993;16(12):1392-1414.

18. Szabo RM, Slater RR, Farver TB, Stanton DB, Sharman WK. The value of diagnostic testing in carpal tunnel syndrome. *J Hand Surg Am.* 1999;24(4):704-714.

19. Wilbourn AJ. The electrodiagnostic examination with peripheral nerve injuries. *Clin Plast Surg.* 2003;30:139-154.

20. Thoma A, Veltri K, Haines T, Duku E. A meta-analysis of randomized controlled trials comparing endoscopic and open carpal tunnel decompression. *Plast Reconstr Surg.* 2004;114(5):1137-1146.

21. Macadam SA, Ghandi R, Bezuhly M, Lefaivre KA. Simple decompression versus anterior subcutaneous and submuscular transposition of the ulnar nerve for cubital tunnel syndrome: a meta-analysis. *J Hand Surg Am.* 2008;33(8):1314.e1-12.

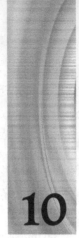

10

COMMON TENDINOPATHIES OF THE WRIST AND ELBOW

David Essig, MD and Seth D. Dodds, MD

INTRODUCTION

Tendinopathies of the wrist and elbow are common conditions that can result in acute or chronic symptoms. They are typically referred to as "overuse syndromes" due to the fact that they are often the result of repetitive motions. Tendinopathy occurs when the stress sustained on a tendon surpasses the strength and endurance of the tissue. While tendinopathies have classically been referred to as "tendonitis," it is rarely the case that inflammatory cells are present within

Culp RW, Jacoby SM. *Musculoskeletal Examination of the Elbow, Wrist, and Hand: Making the Complex Simple* (pp. 212-227). © 2012 Taylor & Francis Group.

the tendon itself. Rather, tendinopathies of the upper extremity are usually the result of either tendonitis or paratendonitis.[1]

Tendinosis is the result of intratendinous degeneration and can be the result of aging, microtrauma, and vascular compromise.[2] Histologically, it is characterized by collagen disorganization and an increase in mucoid ground substance.[3] Lateral epicondylitis is an example of a tendonitis. On the other hand, paratendonitis is the inflammation of the surrounding paratenon typically caused by the friction of tendon excursion over a bony prominence or within a compartment. There can be a mononuclear infiltrate with fibrinous exudates associated with paratendonitis. This entity is distinct from proliferative tenosynovitis (or infectious tenosynovitis), which is characterized by significant synovitis and inflammation.

Tendinosis and paratendonitis can occur in conjunction with one another. For example, the stenosing tendovaginitis of a trigger finger or de Quervain's disease may be initiated by a paratendonitis of the flexor tendons or simply by the attritional wear of a tendon as it courses within a narrowly constricted fibro-osseous tunnel. Stenosing tendovaginitis can progress to a degenerative tendonitis of the affected flexor tendons as fibrocartilaginous metaplasia and thickening occurs within the tendon sheath.

Some of the more common tendinopathies of the wrist include de Quervain's disease, intersection syndrome, and flexor carpi radialis (FCR) tendinopathy, while those of the elbow include lateral and medial epicondylitis. While their prevalence and treatment varies, the general approach is nonsurgical with activity modifications followed by more aggressive therapies for refractory cases (Table 10-1).

DE QUERVAIN'S DISEASE

History

Fritz de Quervain was the first to describe stenosing tendovaginitis of the first dorsal compartment in a case series in 1895.[4] However, it was not until 1936 that the condition became known as de Quervain's disease. Finkelstein was the first individual to describe a specific physical exam test for the

Table 10-1

Helpful Hints

	Anatomic Location	History	Physical Exam	Nonoperative Management	Surgical Treatment
de Quervain's disease	First dorsal compartment	Radial-sided wrist pain with grasping and lifting	First dorsal compartment tenderness and positive Finkelstein's test	Thumb spica splinting, corticosteroid injection	Surgical release of the first dorsal compartment
Intersection syndrome	Second dorsal compartment	Dorsal wrist pain with pulling and twisting	Dorsal wrist pain with resisted wrist extension and rotation	Splinting in wrist extension, NSAIDs, activity modification, corticosteroid injections	Surgical release of the second dorsal compartment
FCR tendonitis	FCR tendon	Volar forearm pain with resisted wrist flexion	Pain with resisted wrist flexion	Physical therapy, NSAIDs, corticosteroid injections, wrist splint	Surgical release of the FCR tendon sheath
Lateral epicondylitis	Lateral epicondyle	Lateral forearm pain with resisted wrist extension and lifting with a pronated forearm	Cozen's test, chair pick-up test	Activity modification, counterforce brace, corticosteroid injections, strengthening of wrist and digital extensors	Open or arthroscopic release, and débridement of degenerative tendon
Medial epicondylitis	Medial epicondyle	Forearm pain with resisted probation and wrist flexion	Tenderness over anterior medial epicondyle	Open or arthroscopic release, and débridement of degenerative tendon	Open release and débridement of degenerative tendon

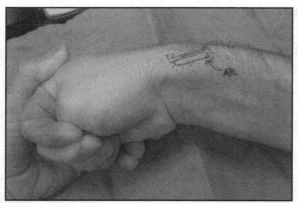

Figure 10-1. The Eichoff maneuver. The patient grasps his or her own thumb, and the examiner deviates the wrist ulnarly.

diagnosis of de Quervain's disease. Clinically, patients complain of pain along the radial side of the wrist that increases with grasping and lifting objects. People at risk for developing the disorder are those who perform repetitive lifting tasks with an extended and abducted thumb, such as new parents frequently lifting a newborn baby. Women are more often affected than men.

Examination

On physical examination, there is usually tenderness at the first dorsal compartment over the radial aspect of the radial styloid. Pain may radiate both proximally and distally along the abductor pollicis longus (APL) and the extensor pollicis brevis (EPB), which reside in the first dorsal compartment. The Finkelstein test is pathognomonic for the disease.[5] In this test, the hand and thumb are grasped by the examiner, and the hand and wrist are deviated ulnarly. A positive test reproduces the pain. An alternative test is the Eichoff maneuver in which the patient clenches his or her own thumb in his or her fist and the examiner deviates the hand and wrist ulnarly, reproducing the pain (Figure 10-1). In later stages of de Quervain's disease, triggering of the APL and/or EPB may be palpable with active or passive thumb motion.

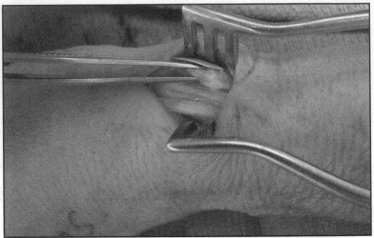

Figure 10-2. This clinical photograph of a de Quervain's release (hand is to the right) shows a thickened first dorsal compartment retinaculum (held by forceps) from fibrocartilaginous metaplasia.

Pathoanatomy

The disease is a result of friction within the first dorsal compartment, which results in hypertrophy and stiffening of the retinaculum. The overall result is increased pressure on the gliding tendons, leading to increased fibrous tissue within the tendon sheaths as well as myxoid degeneration (Figure 10-2).[6] Furthermore, multiple slips of the APL as well as septations within the compartment may contribute to the disease. For example, the EPB is frequently found resting in a separate subsheath within the first dorsal compartment.

Imaging

Routine use of imaging studies is usually not needed because the diagnosis is a clinical one. Plain radiographs, ultrasound, magnetic resonance imaging (MRI), and bone scans have all been used to support the diagnosis. Ultrasound, in particular, has been used to both diagnose and assess treatments.[7] Typical findings include thickening of the retinaculum and irregularities within the tendon sheath.

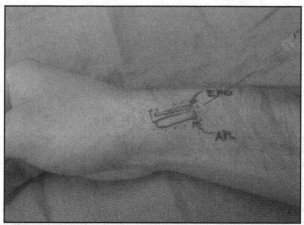

Figure 10-3. Injection of the first dorsal compartment for the treatment of de Quervain's disease.

Treatment

Both conservative and surgical treatments can be used for treatment. Nonsurgical treatments include rest, splinting, activity modification, nonsteroidal anti-inflammatory drugs, and steroid injections. Corticosteroid injections can be highly successful, with rates as high as 80% reported.[4] Failure of injections has been linked to a separate compartment for the EPB tendon. The injection is carried out with the wrist in slight ulnar deviation (Figure 10-3). Using a preferred water-soluble corticosteroid preparation, the injection is performed at the level of the radial styloid. Complications with this procedure include hypopigmentation, subdermal atrophy, and possible tendon rupture.

Surgical procedures for de Quervain's disease have the goal of decompressing the first dorsal compartment. It is important to release any additional slips of the APL and release any additional compartments. It has been found that those who fail to respond to a steroid injection usually have an aberrant compartment.[8] Typical procedures involve an incision over the first dorsal compartment (centered over the radial styloid) with careful dissection down to the compartment to avoid and protect the radial sensory nerve. The extensor retinaculum is incised along its dorsal border, and the compartment

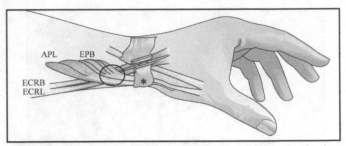

Figure 10-4. Location of intersection syndrome between the first and second dorsal compartments.

is explored with careful attention to any intracompartmental septae that must be removed. After decompression, the skin is closed, and the patient is placed in a thumb spica. Complications that have been reported are those related to injury of the radial sensory nerve, continued pain secondary to incomplete decompression, and volar subluxation of the tendons.

INTERSECTION SYNDROME

Intersection syndrome is a tendinopathy of the second dorsal compartment of the wrist. It was first described by Velpeau in 1841. Symptoms are exacerbated by pulling and twisting motions of the hand, which include radial deviation. Patients who participate in racquet sports and weight lifting are susceptible to this stenosing tendovaginitis.[9]

Examination

The physical exam in intersection syndrome tends to reveal pain and swelling in the proximal part of the forearm. This pain is usually 4 to 8 cm proximal to the radial styloid (Figure 10-4). While no specific diagnostic tests exist, pain is brought on with resisted wrist extension and rotation of the wrist while it is radially deviated.

Pathoanatomy

While the pathophysiology of intersection syndrome has not been fully agreed upon, it is currently believed to be a stenosing tendovaginitis like de Quervain's disease but involving the second dorsal compartment rather than the first.[10] Historically, surgeons believed symptoms were generated by friction between the first and second dorsal compartments that created a bursitis and hypertrophy of the undersurface of the APL tendon, and led to increased pressure on the second dorsal compartment.

Imaging

As intersection syndrome is a clinical diagnosis, there is no preferred imaging test. Plain radiographs may be helpful in ruling out other conditions such as fracture, arthrosis, avascular necrosis, and calcific tendonitis.

Treatment

Treatment of this syndrome tends to be nonoperative. Recommendations include activity modifications, anti-inflammatory medication, ice, hand splints with 15 degrees of wrist extension, and corticosteroid injection into the second dorsal compartment.[11] Surgical options include decompression of the second dorsal compartment in a similar manner to that of decompressing the first dorsal compartment for de Quervain's disease.

Tendinopathy of the Flexor Carpi Radialis

Patients tend to complain of pain with resisted wrist flexion with this tendinopathy. Often, affected individuals are those who play racquet sports, golf, or baseball. The pain is volar and extends from the volar distal pole of the scaphoid proximally along the flexor carpi radialis tendon.

Examination

On exam, pain is often noted on palpation of the insertion of the tendon and with resisted wrist flexion. One physical exam test described by Lister refers to dorsiflexing the relaxed wrist to elicit pain in the region of the insertion of the tendon.[9]

Pathoanatomy

The tendon lays in a fibro-osseous tunnel distally, which transitions to a tendon sheath as the tendon leaves the carpus. Its tendon sheath is separate from and radial to the carpal tunnel. The tendon takes up 90% of its tunnel and sheath width and is susceptible to symptoms associated with pathology of the neighboring carpal structures including scaphoid fractures, scaphoid cysts, arthritis of the scaphoid-trapezium joint, and first carpal-metacarpal arthritis.[12] The tendon also may be affected primarily by tenosynovitis.

Imaging

The diagnosis is clinical, and imaging is not generally beneficial. However, plain radiographs may aid in the diagnosis of associated pathology, if they reveal carpal or metacarpal arthritis or a history of trauma to the scaphoid or distal radius.

Treatment

The management of flexor carpi radialis (FCR) tendinopathy is generally nonoperative as well, including resting, nonsteroidal anti-inflammatory drugs (NSAIDs), splinting, stretching, and steroid injection. For cases resistant to these modalities, operative decompression of the tendon sheath and the distal aspect of the fibro-osseous tunnel may be performed.[13] A volar incision is made, beginning proximal to the wrist crease and extending in a zig-zag fashion to the thenar eminence, as needed. The tendon sheath overlying the FCR is identified and incised longitudinally. If more distal release of the fibro-osseous tunnel is desired, the thenar muscles may be reflected radially off of their origin, and the tunnel is opened in a proximal to distal fashion. Complete release is confirmed by fully mobilizing the tendon from the trapezial groove.

LATERAL EPICONDYLITIS

Commonly referred to as "tennis elbow," patients complain of lateral elbow pain with radiation into the dorsal forearm. Patients are usually between 35 and 50 years of age with men

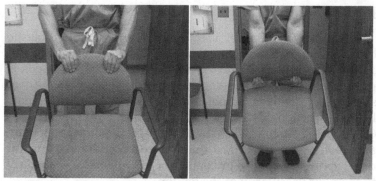

Figure 10-5. Chair pick-up test. With the forearm pronated, a chair is lifted off of the ground, causing pain over the lateral epicondyle. However, when the chair is lifted with the forearm supinated, pain is not produced.

and women being equally affected.[14] Pain is exacerbated by resisted wrist extension, forceful grasp, and lifting with a pronated forearm. Patients also complain of weakness and loss of confidence in the affected arm.

Examination

Tenderness can be elicited on physical exam just distal and anterior to the lateral epicondyle.[14] Pain may also be seen with a maneuver known as Cozen's test, in which the patient's forearm is pronated and pain is elicited with resisted wrist extension.[1] A similar test that succinctly demonstrates to the patient not only the pathoanatomy, but also its essential treatment, is called the chair pick-up test (Figure 10-5). The patient, standing, is asked to pick up a chair by its back with the forearms pronated and the palms down. Typically, pain occurs at the lateral epicondyle, reproducing the patient's symptoms. The chair is returned to the floor. The patient then supinates the forearms, placing the palms up, and lifts the chair again. Typically, there is no pain with supination lifting.

It is important to differentiate lateral epicondylitis from other lateral elbow pathology including posterior interosseous nerve entrapment, lateral collateral ligament strain, intra-articular pathology, synovitis, and fractures.

Pathoanatomy

The disease was first identified as an "angiofibroblastic hyperplasia" of the extensor carpi radialis brevis tendon in 1979.[15] Like other tendinoses, a lack of inflammatory cells is present. In contrast, histologic examination shows the invasion of disorganized fibroblasts as well as vascular elements lacking functionality that are characteristic of degeneration.[16] Overall, the histologic changes disrupt the normal tendon architecture. It is theorized that this reaction may be a result of an aborted response to healing of microtears or secondary to the poor vascularity of the tendon.

Imaging

Plain radiographs are the initial test of choice and may reveal calcific tendonitis of the lateral epicondyle in approximately 7% of patients.[17] However, rarely did the radiographs alter treatment. Ultrasound may also be helpful in that it may reveal calcific tendonitis, tendon thickening, hypoechoic region within the tendon, and bone irregularities.[18] However, while ultrasound has a high sensitivity for detecting lesions in symptomatic epicondylitis, it lacks specificity.

MRI has also demonstrated changes in lateral epicondylitis. Studies have shown increased T1 signal within the tendons, increased fat-saturated FSE sequences, and tendon thickening.[19] Edema has been found in symptomatic individuals but is not specific for the diagnosis.[14]

Treatment

A variety of nonsurgical treatments exist, including splinting, NSAIDs, physical therapy, and injection therapy. Splints that have been used include both wrist and compressive, or counterforce, forearm braces. A wrist orthosis prevents excess strain on the extensor muscles, while counterforce forearm braces attempt to limit muscle belly excursion. Physical therapy treatments include maneuvers such as the Cyriax method, which couples massage with varus force on the elbow.[14] Prospective studies have shown that physical therapy is superior to stand-alone treatment with forearm braces.[20] However, combination therapy failed to provide any added benefit.

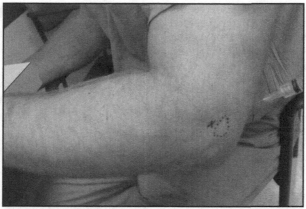

Figure 10-6. Injection for lateral epicondylitis: The injection area is just anterior to the lateral epicondyle and marked by the "X."

Injections have been used for treatment with the mainstay being a combination of local anesthetic and corticosteroid injection (Figure 10-6). One randomized trial comparing corticosteroid injection with NSAID and placebo treatment showed excellent early reduction in pain.[21] However, there was no significant difference among the groups at 1 year.

Various operative interventions have been proposed including open or percutaneous release of the extensor origin, débridement of the extensor origin, anconeus rotation, denervation of the lateral epicondyle, and arthroscopic treatment.[14] Nirschl's classic surgery, later refined to provide for a mini-open technique, involves lifting the extensor carpi radialis longus (ECRL) off of the extensor carpi radialis brevis (ECRB) and débridement of unhealthy tendonitis tissue (Figure 10-7).[16] Nirschl's results included nearly a 98% improvement from preoperative status. These results have not been matched in other studies, nor have meta-analyses of the literature revealed one type of operative procedure to provide superior results over the others.[15,22]

MEDIAL EPICONDYLITIS

This disorder affects the proximal wrist flexors and pronator. It is most prevalent in the fourth and fifth decades of

Figure 10-7. After débridement of degenerative ECRB, the reflected anterior capsule is shown after retraction of the ECRL anteriorly. EDC origin is shown below the exposed capitellum.

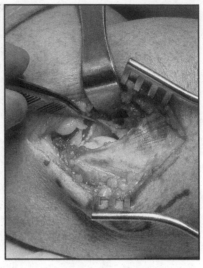

life, affecting men and women equally.[23] The dominant arm is usually affected. Pain may radiate into the forearm and is exacerbated by resisted forearm pronation, resisted wrist flexion, and heavy gripping.[1] It is often seen in throwing athletes but can also affect recreational athletes and manual laborers.

Examination

Patients usually exhibit pain on physical exam approximately 5 mm to 10 mm anterior and distal to the anterior midpoint of the medial epicondyle of the pronator teres and flexor carpi radialis.[23] Pain can usually be elicited with resisted pronation of the forearm with the wrist held in flexion. Occasionally, patients will lack full extension of the affected elbow.[16] It is important to differentiate medial epicondylitis from other elbow pathologies. These include ulnar neuritis and ulnar collateral ligament injury.

Pathoanatomy

Similar to lateral epicondylitis, medial epicondylitis is not the result of an inflammatory process, but rather that of an angiofibroblastic response. Again, the response is believed to be attributed to microtrauma of the flexor carpi radialis and the pronator teres tendons with only a partial reparative response.[23]

Imaging

Similar to lateral epicondylitis, radiographs may reveal calcifications within the tendons in up to 25% of affected individuals. MRI and ultrasound may also be of benefit for analyzing concomitant ulnar collateral injuries. Finally, nerve conduction studies may help in cases of neurologic symptoms to evaluate the ulnar nerve and the possibility of cubital tunnel syndrome.[23]

Treatment

Nonoperative treatment is the primary therapy. Three phases of nonsurgical treatment have been described.[23] The first phase involves activity modification with ice and NSAIDs. In addition, a corticosteroid injection may be employed. However, in a prospective study comparing corticosteroid injection to placebo, there was no difference in symptoms at 1 year.[24] The second phase involves the addition of a regimented exercise regimen to restore strength and flexibility. The final phase seeks to modify the equipment that the patient uses in his or her occupation or sport as well as optimizing the technique so as to minimize the risk of recurrence.

While various surgical techniques have been proposed, they are reserved for those refractory to conservative therapy. Both percutaneous releases and epicondylectomies have been described. However, the ultimate goal is the removal of the diseased, degenerated tendon and the promotion of vascularity to achieve a full healing response. The technique, as described by Nirschl,[1] involves a longitudinal fascial incision from the tip of the medial epicondyle directed distally. Diseased tendon is removed in an elliptical fashion, and the defect is subsequently repaired. Ulnar nerve symptoms should also be addressed, if present. Improvement in pain using this technique approached 85%.[16]

CONCLUSION

While there are a number of different tendinopathies affecting the wrist and elbow, they tend to share similarities with regard to the fact that their etiologies are from repetitive motions, and their pathophysiology is that of a degenerative process. While nonoperative therapy is the mainstay for most tendinopathies, surgical procedures are directed at decompressing the compartment or sheath housing the tendon in cases of stenosing tendovaginitis or removing degenerated tendon at the bony origin of muscles in cases of tendonitis. While the currently described surgical procedures provide good to excellent results in those patients refractory to conservative therapy, future directions may include less invasive techniques as well as biologic growth factors to promote tendon healing and vascularity.

REFERENCES

1. Wainstein JL, Nailor TE. Tendinitis and tendinosis of the elbow, wrist, and hands. *Clin Occup Environ Med.* 2006;5(2):299-322.
2. Maffulli N, Wong J, Almekinders, LC. Types and epidemiology of tendinopathy. *Clin Sports Med.* 2003;22(4):675-692.
3. Khan KM, Cook JL, Bonar F, Harcourt P, Astrom M. Histopathology of common tendinopathies. Update and implications for clinical management. *Sports Med.* 1999;27(6):393-408.
4. Ilyas AM, Ast M, Schaffer AA, Thoder J. De quervain tenosynovitis of the wrist. *J Am Acad Orthop Surg.* 2007;15(12):757-764.
5. Finkelstein H. Stenosing tendovaginitis at the radial styloid process. *J Bone Joint Surg Am.* 1930;12:509-540.
6. Clarke MT, Lyall HA, Grant JW, Mattewson MH. The histopathology of de Quervain's disease. *J Hand Surg Br.* 1998;23(6):732-734.
7. Giovagnorio F, Andreoli C, De Cicco ML. Ultrasonographic evaluation of de Quervain disease. *J Ultrasound Med.* 1997;16(10):685-689.
8. Harvey FJ, Harvey PM, Horsley MW. De Quervain's disease: surgical or nonsurgical treatment. *J Hand Surg Am.* 1990;15(1):83-87.
9. Rettig AC. Wrist and hand overuse syndromes. *Clin Sports Med.* 2001;20(3):591-611.
10. Grundberg AB, Reagan DS. Pathologic anatomy of the forearm: intersection syndrome. *J Hand Surg Am.* 1985;10(2):299-302.
11. Pantukosit S, Petchkrua W, Stiens SA. Intersection syndrome in Buriram Hospital: a 4-yr prospective study. *Am J Phys Med Rehabil.* 2001;80(9):656-661.
12. Bishop AT, Gabel G, Carmichael SW. Flexor carpi radialis tendinitis. Part I: Operative anatomy. *J Bone Joint Surg Am.* 1994;76(7):1009-1014.
13. Gabel G, Bishop AT, Wood MB. Flexor carpi radialis tendinitis. Part II: Results of operative treatment. *J Bone Joint Surg Am.* 1994;76(7):1015-1018.
14. Faro F, Wolf JM. Lateral epicondylitis: review and current concepts. *J Hand Surg Am.* 2007;32(8):1271-1279.

15. Nirschl RP, Pettrone FA. Tennis elbow. The surgical treatment of lateral epicondylitis. *J Bone Joint Surg Am.* 1979;61(6A):832-839.
16. Nirschl RP, Ashman ES. Elbow tendinopathy: tennis elbow. *Clin Sports Med.* 2003;22(4):813-836.
17. Pomerance J. Radiographic analysis of lateral epicondylitis. *J Shoulder Elbow Surg.* 2002;11(2):156-157.
18. Levin D, Nazarian LN, Miller TT, et al. Lateral epicondylitis of the elbow: US findings. *Radiology.* 2005;237(1):230-234.
19. Martin CE, Schweitzer ME. MR imaging of epicondylitis. *Skeletal Radiol.* 1998;27(3):133-138.
20. Struijs PA, Kerkhoffs, GM, Assendelft WJ, Van Kijk CN. Conservative treatment of lateral epicondylitis: brace versus physical therapy or a combination of both-a randomized clinical trial. *Am J Sports Med.* 2004;32(2):462-469.
21. Hay EM, Paterson SM, Lewis M, Hoise G, Croft P. Pragmatic randomised controlled trial of local corticosteroid injection and naproxen for treatment of lateral epicondylitis of elbow in primary care. *BMJ.* 1999;319(7215):964-968.
22. Lo MY, Safran MR. Surgical treatment of lateral epicondylitis: a systematic review. *Clin Orthop Relat Res.* 2007;463:98-106.
23. Ciccotti MC, Schwartz MA, Ciccotti MG. Diagnosis and treatment of medial epicondylitis of the elbow. *Clin Sports Med.* 2004;23(4):693-705.
24. Stahl S, Kaufman T. The efficacy of an injection of steroids for medial epicondylitis. A prospective study of sixty elbows. *J Bone Joint Surg Am.* 1997;79(11):1648-1652.

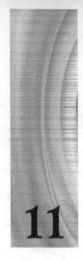

11

ULNAR WRIST
TRIANGULAR FIBROCARTILAGE COMPLEX AND DISTAL RADIO-ULNAR JOINT

Min Jung Park, MD, MMSc and Jeffrey Yao, MD

INTRODUCTION

Ulnar-sided wrist pain may be a difficult entity to diagnose and treat. Acute ulnar-sided wrist pain is typically associated with trauma, and chronic ulnar-sided wrist pain is often associated with repetitive loading. Regardless of the nature and cause, pain in this area of the wrist may be disabling and may significantly affect quality of life. Often, injuries to the triangular fibrocartilage complex (TFCC) with associated instability or other pathology of the distal radioulnar joint

Culp RW, Jacoby SM. *Musculoskeletal Examination of the Elbow, Wrist, and Hand: Making the Complex Simple* (pp. 228-251). © 2012 Taylor & Francis Group.

(DRUJ) are the cause of ulnar-sided wrist pain.[1] The individual components of the TFCC are the articular disk, the palmar and dorsal radioulnar ligaments, the ulnar collateral ligament, and the subsheath of the extensor carpi ulnaris (ECU) tendon.[2] This complex structure confers stability and supports dynamic motion at the DRUJ.

The DRUJ is the distal link between the radius and ulna, and it allows the radius and attached carpus to pivot smoothly around the ulna. The TFCC provides a suspensory mechanism for the carpal bones on the ulnar side of the wrist at the DRUJ. The TFCC also plays a pivotal role in transmission of axial loads at the joint, which makes powerful grip possible.[3] Because the TFCC plays a vital role in stabilizing the DRUJ, it is important to recognize a potential TFCC injury along with DRUJ pathology when evaluating patients with ulnar-sided wrist pain. Although there are a number of other pathologic entities included in the differential diagnosis of ulnar-sided wrist pain including lunotriquetral (LT) instability, injury or tendinosis of the flexor tendon, and ulnar-carpal abutment, a detailed history, physical examination, appropriate imaging, and sound clinical suspicion should enable hand surgeons to recognize the correct pathology.[1]

PATHOANATOMY

DRUJ instability may occur as a result of developmental abnormalities, Madelung's deformity, Essex-Lopresti lesions, inflammatory arthropathies, trauma such as distal radius fracture, or surrounding soft-tissue injuries.[1,4] Fractures of the distal radius are the most common cause of DRUJ instability. Associated ulnar styloid fractures are another common cause of DRUJ instability, with higher likelihood with displacement of greater than 2 mm, but overall functional outcome is not affected by the degree of the ulnar styloid displacement if the distal radius is appropriately fixed.[5] Galeazzi fractures within 7.5 cm of the articular surface frequently result in an unstable DRUJ as well.[6,7] DRUJ dislocations are classified based on the position of the ulna with respect to the radius. Chronic DRUJ instability is often a result of distal radius malunions with either radial shortening or dorsal angulation of the distal radius. The skeletal anatomy of the DRUJ provides little inherent stability to the articulation between the distal radius and ulna. Approximately 80% of load bearing is directed from the carpus to the distal radius and the remaining 20% toward the distal ulna, but positive ulnar variance leads to a significant increase in the load transmitted on the ulnar side.[8] This increased load may lead to ulnar impaction syndrome and increases the risk of a TFCC injury. Patients with ulnar negative variance have been shown to have thicker articular disks.[9] The sigmoid notch is shallow, with approximately 50% greater radius of curvature compared to the ulnar head. At the midrange of motion, 40% to 60% of the articular surface of the ulnar head is seated within the sigmoid notch, but less than 10% is seated at the extremes of pronation and supination.[6,10] The extremes of forearm rotation also result in a relative change of the length of the radius compared to the ulna. With full pronation, the radius is relatively shorter, and at full supination, the radius is relatively longer compared to the ulna. With dynamic pronation and supination of the forearm, one may observe the piston-type motion of the ulna in relation to the radius.[11] One should be familiar with this motion about the sigmoid notch and consider the effects of fixation of the joint during stabilization procedures.

The TFCC is the major stabilizer of the DRUJ. The vascular supply to the TFCC is limited only to the periphery, which explains the poor healing potential of the central disk.[12] The major blood supply of the TFCC arises from the terminal portions of the anterior and posterior interosseous arteries. The TFCC consists of the fibrocartilaginous disk, which is the primary load-bearing component, and the surrounding ligaments that stabilize the DRUJ. The distal radioulnar ligaments are crucial structures in terms of maintaining DRUJ stability. The palmar distal radioulnar ligament is taut in supination, while the dorsal distal radioulnar ligament is taut in pronation. The palmar lip of the sigmoid notch exhibits an osteo-cartilaginous augmentation, which prevents volar subluxation of the ulna, which may be compromised by fracture of the volar distal radius or disruption of the palmar distal radioulnar ligament. TFCC injuries are a frequent cause of ulnar-sided wrist pain, and untreated TFCC injuries may lead to chronic wrist pain and, eventually, DRUJ instability and arthritis.[13]

Table 11-1

Helpful Hints: Palmer Classification

TYPE 1—TRAUMATIC LESION	DESCRIPTION	TYPE 2—DEGENERATIVE LESION	DESCRIPTION
1A	Central disk injury only	2A	TFCC wear
1B	Ulnar-sided peripheral tear of TFCC ± ulnar styloid fracture	2B	TFCC wear with lunate ± ulnar chondromalacia
1C	Distal TFCC disruption	2C	TFCC perforation with lunate ± ulnar chondromalacia
1D	Radial TFCC disruption ± sigmoid notch fracture	2D	TFCC perforation with lunate ± ulnar chondromalacia and lunotriquetral ligament perforation
		2E	TFCC perforation with lunate ± ulnar chondromalacia and lunotriquetral ligament perforation and ulnocarpal arthritis

According to the Palmer classification (Table 11-1), TFCC tears are divided into 2 categories based on their etiology, either traumatic or degenerative.[14] The traumatic type is further classified by their anatomic location as central perforations, ulnar avulsions, distal avulsions, and radial avulsions.

Class 1A (central perforation) represents tears or perforations of the horizontal portion of the TFCC, usually occurring as a 1-mm to 2-mm slit and located 2 to 3 mm medial to the radial attachment of the TFCC. Class 1B (ulnar avulsion) represents a traumatic avulsion of the TFCC from its insertion into the distal portion of the ulna, occasionally with an associated fracture of the base of the styloid process. This lesion is considered unstable. Class 1C represents a distal avulsion of the TFCC at its site of attachment to the lunate or triquetrum, reflective of a tear of the ulnolunate or ulnotriquetral ligaments. A class 1D lesion represents avulsion of the TFCC from its attachment to the radius at the distal aspect of the sigmoid notch, which may be associated with an avulsion fracture of this region.

Degenerative TFCC lesions are caused by progressive stages of ulnocarpal impaction. Most patients over the age of 50 years demonstrate some degree of the TFCC perforation. Palmer Class 2A is TFCC wear from the undersurface, occurring in the central horizontal portion, without perforation. Class 2B is TFCC wear with ulnolunate chondromalacia. The cartilage changes occur on the inferomedial aspect of the lunate or on the more radial portion of the head of the ulna. Class 2C is a TFCC perforation with ulnolunate chondromalacia. The perforation is in the central, horizontal portion of the TFCC and occurs in a more ulnar location than that seen with the traumatic injury that occurs in this zone (Class 1A). Class 2D is a TFCC perforation in the central horizontal portion, associated with ulnolunate arthritis as denoted in 2C, and lunotriquetral ligament perforation. Class 2E is all of the above pathology with ulnocarpal and distal radioulnar degenerative arthritis.[14] Due to repetitive loading of the TFCC, central defects of the articular disk may occur without symptoms. Tears that involve the ligamentous portion of the TFCC or involve a flap that interposes into the joint are likely to result in continued pain despite nonoperative treatment.

DIAGNOSIS

History

Standard questions such as hand dominance, occupation, mechanism of injury, duration of symptoms, and exacerbating factors should be explored thoroughly. Frequently, the mechanism of injury may lead to the accurate diagnosis of the underlying pathology.

Acute peripheral TFCC tears may occur with trauma, typically an acute rotational injury or an axial load to the outstretched and pronated arm.[14,15] Ulnar impaction syndrome may occur due to intrinsic ulnar-positive variance or any kind of traumatic insult that may lead to ulnar-positive variance. Common causes include distal radius fractures and injuries to the radial head.[1] Patients with persistent ulnar-sided wrist pain should be asked thoroughly about their prior injury history. If there is a disruption of the DRUJ, patients may report feeling and/or hearing a popping sensation, and an obvious deformity of the wrist may be observed.

Chronic ulnar-sided wrist pain may also be the result of acute trauma sustained in the past, injuries to neighboring joints, or systemic inflammatory disease, such as rheumatoid arthritis or pseudogout.[1] Therefore, a detailed past medical history and family history should be obtained during the initial consultation. Chronic overuse injuries may also lead to ECU and/or flexor carpi ulnaris (FCU) tendonitis. Lastly, chronic ulnar-sided wrist pain may be due to ulnar impaction syndrome with or without a concomitant degenerative TFCC tear. These patients typically have a long history of indolent ulnar-sided wrist pain and may or may not report a recent change in work habits or sporting activity that require significant change in their use of the wrist joint.

Physical Examination

A good physical examination serves as a link between the patient's subjective complaints and the pathology of the underlying symptoms (Table 11-2). Prior to the examination of the wrist, it is important to inspect the entire upper extremity, including the cervical spine. Any signs of extrinsic etiology of the wrist pain should be further evaluated when necessary. Typically, patients would have no problem localizing pain toward the ulnar side of their wrist when there is underlying pathology. Ideally, a patient's elbow should rest on an examination table in the most comfortable position, so that the examiner has easy access to the wrist. One should carefully look for prior surgical incisions over the wrist, forearm, and elbow. All physical exam findings should be compared with the contralateral side, as some findings may be symmetrical.

Significant swelling on the ulnar side of the wrist is only expected in the setting of the acute fracture or dislocation. The ulnar head is the rounded prominence at the distal end

Table 11-2

Methods for Examination

EXAMINATION	TECHNIQUE	ILLUSTRATION	SIGNIFICANCE
Piano key test	With the radius stabilized, the ulnar head is forced to subluxate/dislocate volar or dorsal with the care taken to examine the possible instability throughout the forearm range of motion in supination and pronation.	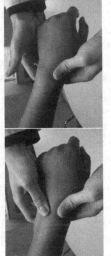	Can be used preoperative or intraoperatively to assess DRUJ instability.
Ulnocarpal stress test	Also known as the TFCC grind test, ulnar deviation and axial loads of patient's wrist while performing forearm pronation and supination reproduces ulnar-sided wrist discomfort.	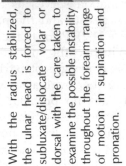	Although not specific, it is a sensitive test for ulnar-sided wrist pathology such as TFCC tear.

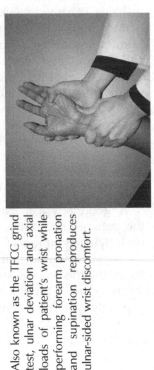

(continued)

Table 11-2 (continued)

Methods for Examination

EXAMINATION	TECHNIQUE	ILLUSTRATION	SIGNIFICANCE
ECU sublux-ation test	ECU is in the correct position in neutral, but as the wrist is supinated and ulnar deviated, the ECU tendon subluxates, and reproduces pain.	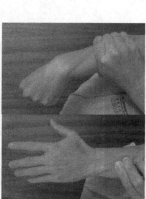	ECU subluxation with ECU sheath disruption can be painful of itself or as TFCC disruption.
Positioning of wrist on x-ray	Shoulder should be abducted 90 degrees with the elbow flexed 90 degrees and the palm of the hand flat on the image intensifier gives the best view of the wrist.	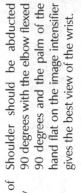	Incorrect placement of the wrist on the image intensifier can give a false sense of DRUJ instability if the wrist is imaged in forearm in supination or pronation, or the beam is directed at an angle due to shoulder/elbow positioning.

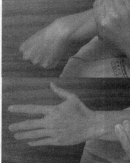

(continued)

Table 11-2 (continued)

Methods for Examination

EXAMINATION	TECHNIQUE	ILLUSTRATION	SIGNIFICANCE
Trampoline test	Intraoperatively, a probe is used to assess the sturdiness of the TFCC by pressing down on the soft tissue.	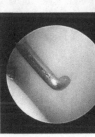	Some bounce back, aka "trampoline effect," is expected from healthy TFCC with tactile sensation of resistance.
Ulnar impaction lesion of lunate	Arthroscopic evaluation of ulnar impaction of lunate.	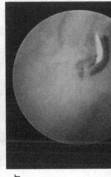	Arthroscopic evaluation of all associated lesions are critical to assess possible etiology of ulnar-sided wrist pain.

of the ulna. It is best examined with the forearm pronated. A dorsally protruding ulnar head that is more prominent than the contralateral side is a sign of a DRUJ injury. Tenderness on palpation in this area may indicate an ulnar styloid fracture or DRUJ instability or arthritis. In order to test for incongruity of the DRUJ, one should use the piano key test, in which the dorsal prominence of the ulnar head is exaggerated following depression and release and with rotation about the wrist joint. Pain and crepitus exacerbated by rotation at the wrist is indicative of arthritic etiology. Alternatively, one may hold the radius in a fixed position and move the distal ulna in volar to dorsal direction. Pain and crepitus should be reproduced at the DRUJ. The ulnar compression test, where the examiner grinds the ulnar head radially against the sigmoid notch, is another useful provocative test that should lead one to suspect DRUJ pathology.[16]

The TFCC is palpated between the ulnar head and the triquetrum along the dorsal-ulnar side of the wrist joint. The fovea should be palpated along the base of the ulnar head and ulnar styloid, and tenderness in this area is defined as the ulnar fovea sign,[17] which is indicative of a TFCC tear or a ulnotriquetral ligament tear. The ulnocarpal stress test (aka, the TFCC grind test) is another test that may help detect a TFCC tear or ulnocarpal abutment. An examiner ulnarly deviates and axially loads the patient's wrist while rotating the forearm. Reproduction of the patient's symptoms is considered a positive test and typically demonstrates pain, clicking, and/or crepitus at the DRUJ. The ulnocarpal stress test is proven to have good sensitivity (89%) in terms of detecting the ulnar-sided wrist pathology.[18] Additionally, disruption of the ulnar extrinsic ligaments of the TFCC may cause volar sag and supination of the ulnar carpus. The relocation test is a provocative test that uses the combined movement of pronation and dorsal translation of the carpus on the ulna, which relocates the carpus into normal alignment. This relocation may confer therapeutic benefit by relieving the wrist pain. Similarly, the pisiform boost test is useful in the setting of ulnocarpal or lunotriquetral instability, as dorsal pressure on the volar pisiform reduces the carpus on the ulna and results in crepitus, clicking, and/or pain. The triquetrum may be palpated along the ulnar border of the wrist with the wrist in radial deviation. It is located just distal to the ulnar styloid

Figure 11-1. LT Ballottement test.

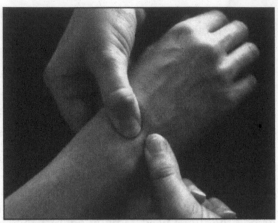

and within the "ulnar snuff box" between the ECU and FCU tendons.[19] Tenderness to palpation in this area is most likely due to fracture or LT instability and may be misinterpreted as a TFCC tear. The LT ballottement test is done by holding the lunate in fixed position and applying dorsal pressure on the pisotriquetral complex, assessing for laxity as the wrist is passively moved radially and ulnarly. A click with pain may be reproduced in patients with an LT injury (Figure 11-1). The ECU tendon courses within the sixth dorsal extensor compartment. It is palpated in the gap between the ulnar styloid and the base of the fifth metacarpal when the forearm is pronated or during active ulnar deviation. Tenderness and pain with resisted ulnar deviation is indicative of ECU pathology. Subluxation caused by a failing ECU subsheath that allows the tendon to bowstring with the wrist in ulnar deviation is best diagnosed with active ulnar deviation in full supination. Selective injections may be helpful in the diagnosis of ulnar-sided wrist pain. Either lidocaine alone or along with a corticosteroid may be used for both diagnostic and therapeutic purposes. Symptom relief after injection into the ECU tendon sheath would localize the symptoms to the ECU tendon.

Imaging

As an initial assessment of ulnar-sided wrist pain, standard radiograph views including posteroanterior (PA), lateral, and oblique views should be obtained. Radiographs will allow one to assess the alignment of the carpus and the DRUJ. Widening on PA views and dorsal or volar displacement on the lateral view is indicative of disruption of the DRUJ. An adequate lateral view is achieved when the pisiform is visualized midway between the volar aspect of the capitate and the distal pole of the scaphoid.[20] Subchondral sclerosis and cystic changes may be evident in cases of ulnocarpal abutment/impaction at the proximal ulnar portion of the lunate and the proximal radial portion of the triquetrum. The 0-degree PA view is of particular importance when evaluating ulnar-sided wrist pathology. The shoulder should be abducted 90 degrees, the elbow flexed 90 degrees, and the hand flat on the x-ray cassette. A good quality PA view is confirmed by visualizing the ECU tendon adjacent to the ulnar styloid, which is directly ulnar and is indicative of neutral wrist position. As discussed previously, ulnar variance may change with forearm rotation, with maximal ulnar positive variance achieved with pronation and forced finger flexion. If ulnar impaction syndrome is suspected, a power-grip PA view should be obtained to evaluate the possible dynamic nature of the pathology.[21,22]

Axial forearm computed tomography (CT) images in pronation and supination may help elucidate dynamic instability of DRUJ that may not be obvious with plain film or clinical exam.[23] The images may also be used to evaluate for possible malunion and arthritic changes of the ulnar head or sigmoid notch. One should take note of the congruency of the ulnar head in the arc of the sigmoid notch of the radius. There are a number of methods that evaluate CT evidence of DRUJ instability, mainly the Mino criteria, the epicenter method, the radioulnar ratio, and the congruency method.[24] The Mino criteria states the ulnar head should be between the line drawn parallel to the dorsal and volar borders of the radius. The test is reported to have a 15% false-positive rate. The radioulnar ratio method is shown to be superior compared to the Mino criteria, the epicenter method, and the congruency method.[24] Contralateral forearm images should be obtained at the same time with the same positions for reference. When using CT images to evaluate DRUJ instability after distal radius fractures, one must be aware that interpretation of the images may be influenced by residual deformities. CT arthrography is useful in detecting scapholunate interosseous ligament (SLIL), lunotriquetral interosseous ligament (LTIL), and central TFCC tears, but not as much for peripheral tears.[25]

The utility of magnetic resonance imaging (MRI) is controversial in the diagnosis of TFCC injuries. Although recent developments in the MR arthrography techniques have shown promising potential, there is no study that shows superiority of MR arthrography over conventional MRI in terms of identifying TFCC injuries.[9] For MRI, patients may be positioned in either the supine or prone position, but prone position using surface coils has been shown to produce better quality images.[26] In order to obtain a diagnostically useful study, a dedicated microscopy wrist coil should be used, and 3 Tesla magnets are preferred over 1.5 Tesla magnets.[27,28]

For patients with ulnar-sided wrist pain, the overall accuracy of MR arthrography in detecting a full-thickness tear of the TFCC is reported to be 79% with a positive predictive value of 0.95, negative predictive value of 0.5, sensitivity of 74%, and specificity of 80%.[29] A negative result of MR arthrography does not confer significant diagnostic value. MRI with intravenous contrast may be useful in the setting of ulnocarpal impaction syndrome or nonunions. Bone hyperemia in the lunate and triquetrum is depicted as low signal density on T1 images and high-density signal in T2 images. If the disease progresses to develop sclerotic changes, both T1 and T2 images would demonstrate low signal density in the area. Triple injection arthrography is a useful study for evaluating the TFCC, the scapholunate ligament, and the LT ligament. Contrast material is injected into the DRUJ, the radiocarpal, and the midcarpal joints. Specific patterns of leakage are observed with different injury patterns. However, many asymptomatic patients may be found to have degenerative tears indicating low specificity.[30,31]

Recently, with the development of better arthroscopic instruments and techniques, arthroscopy is considered the gold standard to identify the above-mentioned lesions, and the procedure may be therapeutic at the same time.[32-34] Through arthroscopy, one can directly detect peripheral tears of the TFCC. Hyperemia along the periphery, tears of the LT ligament, injuries to the ECU sheath, and the loss of resiliency to probing—commonly known as the trampoline test—are the signs of a peripheral TFCC injury.[35]

TREATMENT

Table 11-3 summarizes the treatment algorithm. Acute DRUJ dislocations are classified based on the position of the ulnar relative to the radius. Dorsal dislocations (ulna dorsal) may be treated with closed reduction with the forearm positioned in supination. Palmar dislocation should be treated with immobilization with the forearm in pronation. If there is clinically severe joint instability, or it is recognized late, open repair of the TFCC with DRUJ pinning and possibly DRUJ reconstruction may be indicated.

The treatment strategy of a TFCC injury depends on a detailed history, clinical findings, and imaging studies. For peripheral TFCC tears (Palmer 1B), nonoperative management is the initial treatment unless there is gross instability. If there is gross instability on exam, surgical management may be necessary. There may be a concomitant ulnar styloid fracture present with the TFCC tear that would require open reduction and internal fixation of the fracture along with the TFCC repair. Given its vascularity, most isolated, acute peripheral tears of TFCC are expected to heal with immobilization in a long arm cast to resist forearm rotation for 4 to 6 weeks. Failed conservative treatment would require surgical intervention. Although open surgical repair has been the gold standard in the past, recently, many authors favor arthroscopic repair of peripheral TFCC tears.[32,36,37] Arthroscopic repair generally produces good surgical outcome if performed within 4 months for isolated TFCC tears. Excellent surgical outcome of débridement or repair of TFCC injury is well documented in high-level athletes as well.[18] There is no statistically significant difference in outcome measures between open and arthroscopic TFCC repair.[38] The disadvantages of the past arthroscopic TFCC repairs included extra incisions, prominent subcutaneous suture knots, skin problems secondary to a button tied to skin, and even septic arthritis from prominent buttons and sutures. Recently, all-arthroscopic repair of a peripheral TFCC tear has been introduced, and preliminary results have shown promise (Table 11-4).[37]

Palmer 1C injuries are usually treated nonoperatively.[1,32] If repair is necessary, one should be mindful of ulnar arteries

Table 11-3

Ulnar-Sided Wrist Pain Evaluation Protocol

HISTORY AND PHYSICAL

1. Hand dominance
2. Occupation
3. Mechanism of injury
4. Duration of symptoms
5. Exacerbating factors

TREATMENT ALGORITHM

Duration of Symptoms	Treatment Recommendations	Treatment Pearl
Observation for deformity	Obvious fracture and/or dislocation can be inspected. Careful skin inspection should be performed for open injury as well.	After adequate imaging studies are obtained, closed reduction maneuver should be tried. Any open fractures should be promptly washed out in the operating room setting.
Piano key test	Obvious subluxation of DRUJ may indicate gross ligamentous injury.	In the setting of isolated DRUJ instability/subluxation, immobilization in supination or neutral for approximately 4 weeks may be tried. Most frank dislocations/subluxation are in the setting of other associated fracture/dislocation, and if unstable following fracture fixation, DRUJ should be fixed in the OR setting as well.
Ulnar compression test	Sensitive, but not specific test for ulnar-sided wrist pain.	Most often signifies TFCC injury. Careful examination of radiographic findings and history and physical exam should guide whether other advanced imaging such as MRI or arthroscopic examination is warranted.

(continued)

Table 11-3 (continued)

Ulnar-Sided Wrist Pain Evaluation Protocol

TREATMENT ALGORITHM

Duration of Symptoms	Treatment Recommendations	Treatment Pearl
Less than 6 months of symptoms	Trial of conservative measures are almost always warranted.	About 50% of patients diagnosed with TFCC tear will have symptomatic relief with short-arm cast for 4 to 6 weeks. NSAIDs and activity modifications can be helpful. Steroid injection should be used sparingly, and only when there is evidence of marked inflammation and/or degenerative joint changes.
More than 6 months of symptoms	Diagnostic arthroscopy of the wrist is warranted if failed conservative treatment and appropriate imaging studies are obtained without much elucidation of the possible etiology for ulnar-sided wrist pain.	1. Diagnositc arthroscopy with TFCC débridement or repair +/- ulnar styloid ORIF, +/- DRUJ pinning 2. If DRUJ arthrosis is present: a. Ulnar head resection (Darrach +/- stabilization versus Sauvé-Kapandji versus HIT). b. Implant arthroplasty (hemiarthroplasty versus bipolar).

and nerves in this region. Treatment of Palmer 1D injuries is controversial. There is little if any vascularity in that area. Although repairs of these tears have been described, recently, it has been shown that simple débridement has produced satisfactory results. Central tears of the TFCC (Palmer 1A) need either conservative treatment with immobilization or surgical intervention, with the goal of stabilization of DRUJ and restoration of wrist range of motion. Like Palmer 1D-type

Table 11-4

Methods of Treatment

Technique	How It Is Performed	Illustration	Significance
Inside Out Suture Repair	Peripheral tear of TFCC repaired arthroscopically with sutures	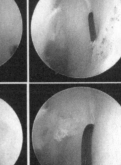	Sutures are brought inside, then knots are tied outside of the TFCC, similar to inside-out meniscal repair technique.
FasT-Fix Meniscal Repair System (Smith and Nephew Endoscopy, Andover, MA)	Alternative method of peripheral TFCC repair using FasT-Fix		All-inside technique without the knot outside of the TFCC for possible subcutaneous irritation.

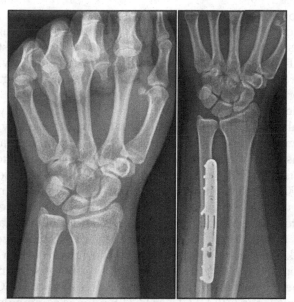

Figure 11-2. Symptomatic ulnar positive variance treated with ulnar shortening osteotomy.

injuries, central tears are unlikely to heal due to the avascular nature of the articular disk. Simple débridement is appropriate, and up to two-thirds of the disk may be debrided without risk of affecting load transfer.[32]

Although ulnar-positive or neutral variance does not need to be simultaneously corrected at the time of arthroscopic repair of peripheral TFCC tears, patients with persistent pain following the repair may benefit from an ulnar shortening procedure (Figure 11-2).[39,40]

In the face of ulnar-neutral or positive variance with significant chondromalacia of the ulnar head or lunate, or any suspicion of ulnar impaction syndrome, one should consider ulnar recession (wafer procedure) or ulnar shortening osteotomy. During the wafer procedure, the distal 2 to 4 mm of ulnar head is resected, with the goal of about 2 mm of ulnar-negative variance postoperatively.[41,42] It may be performed successfully with an arthroscopic approach. Degenerative tears of the TFCC tend to respond poorly to conservative management, and often débridement and/or ulnar shortening osteotomy is necessary, depending on the patient's ulnar variance. Ulnar shortening osteotomies may also be used to successfully treat patients with LTIL tears and early post-traumatic DRUJ arthritis.[43] In cases of DRUJ instability with an irreparable TFCC, reconstruction of the radioulnar ligament is recommended.[10,44]

Patients with chronic untreated DRUJ instability will undoubtedly develop distal radioulnar incongruity with degenerative joint disease. After its introduction by Darrach, various forms of ulnar head resections have been used to treat patients with DRUJ arthritis. During the ulnar head resection, the TFCC are left undisturbed. Approximately 6 to 8 mm of distal ulna is removed, with or without ECU tenodesis or pronator interposition (if needed for each individual case for added stabilization).[45] Patients are usually immobilized for 2 weeks following the procedure. The hemiresection interposition arthroplasty (HIT) described by Bowers[46] can offer therapeutic benefit to the patients with an intact TFCC. The palmaris longus (PL), ECU, or FCU tendon is commonly used as an interposition graft. If the patient has ulnar-positive variance, an ulnar shortening osteotomy should be done before proceeding with the procedure. A matched ulnar resection is another variation of the ulnar head resection, which may be used in the setting of both rheumatoid or post-traumatic DRUJ arthrosis.[47] With this procedure, the resection of the ulnar head is contoured to the radius, instead of the transverse resection of the distal ulna. Despite all the modifications, these procedures do not restore the normal anatomy, and ulnar stump instability has been a frequent problem postoperatively.[45] Excessive resection of the distal ulna may also result in radioulnar impingement. ECU subluxation may be a source of postoperative pain as well as the palmar subluxation or ulnar translation of the carpus. Ulnar head resections should only be done in patients who maintain low demand of their wrist.

The Sauvé-Kapandji procedure is another option for patients with DRUJ instability and/or arthritis.[4] The procedure fuses the distal radius to the distal ulna at the radiocarpal joint after resection of a 1-cm cuff of the ulnar shaft. The distal ulna is positioned proximally to be ulnar neutral after the resection of the ulnar shaft. The pronator quadratus or a soft tissue sleeve may be used to fill the void created by

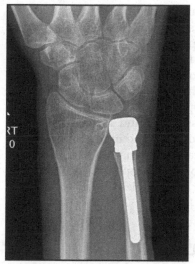

Figure 11-3. Ulnar head arthroplasty.

the ulnar shaft resection.[4] The procedure takes advantage of the intact TFCC and confers several advantages compared to ulnar head resection techniques. With the Sauvé-Kapandji technique, one maintains the uninterrupted articular surface for the proximal carpal articulation with normal contour of the ulnar head. This creates better physiologic load transmission to the forearm. The use of pronator quadratus and/or ECU to stabilize the ulnar stump can also prevent potential dislocation. As with the ulnar head resection procedures, the Sauvé-Kapandji procedure is not designed to provide a very durable DRUJ joint that can withstand heavy labor. The proximal ulna may become unstable and cause pain in some patients, and synostosis at the osteotomy site is another source of potential complication.

The idea of implant arthroplasty of the DRUJ has been gaining interest as of late.[48] Hemiarthroplasty (distal ulna replacement) implants have been available (Figure 11-3), but they have not been shown to offer much benefit compared to the variations of resection arthroplasties or the Sauvé-Kapandji procedures.[48] Bipolar DRUJ replacement implants are thought to provide enough stability at the DRUJ while preserving enough of the native motion at the joint. The semi-constrained construct allows the migration of the radius with forearm supination and pronation. The bipolar prosthesis is reported to be used in patients with failed ulnar head resections or hemi-arthroplasty. A proximal ulnar length of 11 cm is required to be a candidate for the bipolar prosthesis, and patients who have had the bipolar prosthesis as their primary procedure have done better than the others.[48] Patients who underwent the bipolar arthroplasty of the DRUJ have been reported to have better grip strength and restoration of the lifting motion at the joint.[49] However, the inherent instability of the DRUJ coupled with great forces that involve that joint may lead to premature wear of these implants. More longer-term studies are needed prior to the widespread acceptance and use of these implants.

CONCLUSION

Ulnar-sided wrist pain is a common entity and may be difficult to treat. Correctly identifying the underlying pathology is challenging, and offering the most appropriate treatment option for each individual patient may be even more difficult. Early identification of symptoms and intervention may greatly reduce future morbidity for patients by allowing the use of less invasive treatment modalities. The advancement in diagnostic imaging such as MRI, arthrography, and arthroscopy will certainly enable health care providers to better recognize pathology. Hand and orthopedic surgeons should have a concrete knowledge of how to obtain a detailed history and physical exam, in conjunction with the latest improvements in arthroscopic repair techniques and DRUJ arthroplasty implants in order to allow the patients with challenging TFCC and/or DRUJ injuries to achieve pain relief and regain the motion and the strength to carry out activities of daily life.

REFERENCES

1. Sachar K. Ulnar-sided wrist pain: evaluation and treatment of triangular fibrocartilage complex tears, ulnocarpal impaction syndrome, and lunotriquetral ligament tears. *J Hand Surg [Am]*. 2008;33:1669-1679.
2. Palmer AK, Werner FW. The triangular fibrocartilage complex of the wrist—anatomy and function. *J Hand Surg [Am]*. 1981;6:153-162.

3. Haugstvedt JR, Berger RA, Nakamura T, Neale P, Berglund L, An KN. Relative contributions of the ulnar attachments of the triangular fibrocartilage complex to the dynamic stability of the distal radioulnar joint. *J Hand Surg [Am]*. 2006;31:445-451.

4. Slater RR Jr. The Sauvé-Kapandji procedure. *J Hand Surg [Am]*. 2008;33:1632-1638.

5. Souer JS, Ring D, Matschke S, Audige L, Marent-Huber M, Jupiter JB. Effect of an unrepaired fracture of the ulnar styloid base on outcome after plate-and-screw fixation of a distal radial fracture. *J Bone Joint Surg Am*. 2009;91:830-838.

6. Szabo RM. Distal radioulnar joint instability. *J Bone Joint Surg Am*. 2006;88:884-894.

7. Rettig ME, Raskin KB. Galeazzi fracture-dislocation: a new treatment-oriented classification. *J Hand Surg [Am]*. 2001;26:228-235.

8. Palmer AK. The distal radioulnar joint. Anatomy, biomechanics, and triangular fibrocartilage complex abnormalities. *Hand Clin*. 1987;3:31-40.

9. Yoshioka H, Tanaka T, Ueno T, et al. Study of ulnar variance with high-resolution MRI: correlation with triangular fibrocartilage complex and cartilage of ulnar side of wrist. *J Magn Reson Imaging*. 2007;26:714-719.

10. Lawler E, Adams BD. Reconstruction for DRUJ instability. Hand (N Y). 2007;2:123-126.

11. Yeh GL, Beredjiklian PK, Katz MA, Steinberg DR, Bozentka DJ. Effects of forearm rotation on the clinical evaluation of ulnar variance. *J Hand Surg [Am]*. 2001;26:1042-1046.

12. Thiru RG, Ferlic DC, Clayton ML, McClure DC. Arterial anatomy of the triangular fibrocartilage of the wrist and its surgical significance. *J Hand Surg [Am]*. 1986;11:258-263.

13. Ward LD, Ambrose CG, Masson MV, Levaro F. The role of the distal radioulnar ligaments, interosseous membrane, and joint capsule in distal radioulnar joint stability. *J Hand Surg [Am]*. 2000;25:341-351.

14. Palmer AK. Triangular fibrocartilage complex lesions: a classification. *J Hand Surg [Am]*. 1989;14:594-606.

15. Viegas SF, Patterson RM, Hokanson JA, Davis J. Wrist anatomy: incidence, distribution, and correlation of anatomic variations, tears, and arthrosis. *J Hand Surg [Am]*. 1993;18:463-475.

16. Rettig AC. Athletic injuries of the wrist and hand. Part I: traumatic injuries of the wrist. *Am J Sports Med*. 2003;31:1038-1048.

17. Tay SC, Tomita K, Berger RA. The "ulnar fovea sign" for defining ulnar wrist pain: an analysis of sensitivity and specificity. *J Hand Surg [Am]*. 2007;32:438-444.

18. Nakamura R, Horii E, Imaeda T, Nakao E, Kato H, Watanabe K. The ulnocarpal stress test in the diagnosis of ulnar-sided wrist pain. *J Hand Surg [Br]*. 1997;22:719-723.

19. Beckenbaugh RD. Accurate evaluation and management of the painful wrist following injury. An approach to carpal instability. *Orthop Clin North Am*. 1984;15:289-306.

20. May O. [The pisiform bone: sesamoid or carpal bone?]. *Ann Chir Main Memb Super*. 1996;15:265-271.

21. Tomaino MM. The importance of the pronated grip x-ray view in evaluating ulnar variance. *J Hand Surg [Am]*. 2000;25:352-357.

22. Tomaino MM, Rubin DA. The value of the pronated-grip view radiograph in assessing dynamic ulnar positive variance: a case report. *Am J Orthop*. 1999;28:180-181.

23. Nakamura T, Nakao Y, Ikegami H, Sato K, Takayama S. Open repair of the ulnar disruption of the triangular fibrocartilage complex with double three-dimensional mattress suturing technique. *Tech Hand Up Extrem Surg*. 2004;8:116-123.

24. Lo IK, MacDermid JC, Bennett JD, Bogoch E, King GJ. The radioulnar ratio: a new method of quantifying distal radioulnar joint subluxation. *J Hand Surg [Am]*. 2001;26:236-243.

25. Bille B, Harley B, Cohen H. A comparison of CT arthrography of the wrist to findings during wrist arthroscopy. *J Hand Surg [Am]*. 2007;32:834-841.

26. Bittersohl B, Huang T, Schneider E, et al. High-resolution MRI of the triangular fibrocartilage complex (TFCC) at 3T: comparison of surface coil and volume coil. *J Magn Reson Imaging*. 2007;26:701-707.

27. Saupe N, Prussmann KP, Luechinger R, Bosiger P, Marincek B, Weishaupt D. MR imaging of the wrist: comparison between 1.5- and 3-T MR imaging--preliminary experience. *Radiology*. 2005;234:256-264.

28. Tanaka T, Yoshioka H, Ueno T, Shindo M, Ochiai N. Comparison between high-resolution MRI with a microscopy coil and arthroscopy in triangular fibrocartilage complex injury. *J Hand Surg [Am]*. 2006;31:1308-1314.

29. Joshy S, Lee K, Deshmukh SC. Accuracy of direct magnetic resonance arthrography in the diagnosis of triangular fibrocartilage complex tears of the wrist. *Int Orthop*. 2008;32(2):251-253.

30. Cerezal L, del Pinal F, Abascal F. MR imaging findings in ulnar-sided wrist impaction syndromes. *Magn Reson Imaging Clin N Am*. 2004;12:281-299, vi.

31. Cerezal L, del Pinal F, Abascal F, Garcia-Valtuille R, Pereda T, Canga A. Imaging findings in ulnar-sided wrist impaction syndromes. *Radiographics*. 2002;22:105-121.

32. Slutsky DJ, Nagle DJ. Wrist arthroscopy: current concepts. *J Hand Surg [Am]*. 2008;33:1228-1244.

33. Nagle DJ, Benson LS. Wrist arthroscopy: indications and results. *Arthroscopy*. 1992;8:198-203.

34. Chung KC, Zimmerman NB, Travis MT. Wrist arthrography versus arthroscopy: a comparative study of 150 cases. *J Hand Surg [Am]*. 1996;21:591-594.

35. Hermansdorfer JD, Kleinman WB. Management of chronic peripheral tears of the triangular fibrocartilage complex. *J Hand Surg [Am]*. 1991;16:340-346.

36. Yao J. All-arthroscopic triangular fibrocartilage complex repair: safety and biomechanical comparison with a traditional outside-in technique in cadavers. *J Hand Surg [Am]*. 2009;34:671-676.

37. Yao J, Dantuluri P, Osterman AL. A novel technique of all-inside arthroscopic triangular fibrocartilage complex repair. *Arthroscopy*. 2007;23:1357 e1-4.

38. Anderson ML, Larson AN, Moran SL, Cooney WP, Amrami KK, Berger RA. Clinical comparison of arthroscopic versus open repair of triangular fibrocartilage complex tears. *J Hand Surg [Am]*. 2008;33:675-682.

39. Reiter A, Wolf MB, Schmid U, et al. Arthroscopic repair of Palmer 1B triangular fibrocartilage complex tears. *Arthroscopy*. 2008;24:1244-1250.

40. Wolf MB, Kroeber MW, Reiter A, et al. Ulnar shortening after TFCC suture repair of Palmer type 1B lesions. *Arch Orthop Trauma Surg*. 2010;130(3):301-306.

41. Feldon P, Terrono AL, Belsky MR. Wafer distal ulna resection for triangular fibrocartilage tears and/or ulna impaction syndrome. *J Hand Surg [Am]*. 1992;17:731-737.

42. Feldon P, Terrono AL, Belsky MR. The "wafer" procedure. Partial distal ulnar resection. *Clin Orthop Relat Res*. 1992:124-129.

43. Scheker LR, Severo A. Ulnar shortening for the treatment of early post-traumatic osteoarthritis at the distal radioulnar joint. *J Hand Surg [Br]*. 2001;26:41-44.

44. Adams BD, Lawler E. Chronic instability of the distal radioulnar joint. *J Am Acad Orthop Surg*. 2007;15:571-575.

45. Lee SK, Hausman MR. Management of the distal radioulnar joint in rheumatoid arthritis. *Hand Clin*. 2005;21:577-589.

46. Bowers WH. Distal radioulnar joint arthroplasty: the hemiresection-interposition technique. *J Hand Surg [Am]*. 1985;10:169-178.

47. Watson HK, Gabuzda GM. Matched distal ulna resection for post-traumatic disorders of the distal radioulnar joint. *J Hand Surg [Am]*. 1992;17:724-730.

48. Scheker LR. Implant arthroplasty for the distal radioulnar joint. *J Hand Surg [Am]*. 2008;33:1639-1644.

49. Laurentin-Perez LA, Goodwin AN, Babb BA, Scheker LR. A study of functional outcomes following implantation of a total distal radioulnar joint prosthesis. *J Hand Surg Eur Vol*. 2008;33:18-28.

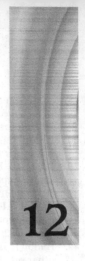

12

ARTHRITIS OF THE ELBOW, WRIST, AND HAND

Brian D. Adams, MD

INTRODUCTION

Arthritis is a broad descriptive term for inflammation and possible damage to joints due to a variety of possible etiologies. Clinically, it is characterized by joint pain, tenderness, limitation of movement, crepitus, effusion, and variable degrees of inflammation. Osteoarthritis (OA), sometimes termed *degenerative arthritis*, is the most common type. Other types result from infection, metabolic conditions, skeletal dysplasias, trauma and inflammatory arthritides (eg, rheumatoid

Culp RW, Jacoby SM. *Musculoskeletal Examination of the Elbow, Wrist, and Hand: Making the Complex Simple* (pp. 252-273). © 2012 Taylor & Francis Group.

arthritis [RA] and psoriatic arthritis), crystalline deposition disease, and neuropathic disorders.[1]

The hand, wrist, and elbow can be affected by all forms of arthritis to varying degrees. In the hand, the joints most frequently affected by OA are the distal interphalangeal (DIP) joints and thumb carpometacarpal (CMC) joint.[2] The metacarpophalangeal (MCP) joints are less commonly affected by OA, but are frequently involved in RA. In the wrist, degenerative arthritis and trauma can cause carpal instability and altered kinematics, resulting in specific patterns of radiocarpal arthritis, which typically first involves the radial scaphoid joint. In advanced RA, wrist deformity can be severe, resulting in secondary loss of hand function. The distal radioulnar joint (DRUJ) is involved occasionally in OA but frequently in RA. The DRUJ deformity resulting from RA is termed the "caput ulna syndrome," in which the ulnar head is subluxated and prominent dorsally. Primary OA of the elbow is rare and most frequently seen in middle-aged male laborers. More common causes of elbow arthritis are post-traumatic, crystalline deposition, inflammation, osteonecrosis, and osteochondritis dissecans. Elbow involvement has been reported in up to 65% of patients with RA, but hand and wrist involvement is usually more disabling early in the disease.

HISTORY

Symptoms of arthritis usually develop slowly but are progressive, causing the patient intermittent pain, stiffness, and weakness. Pain is exacerbated by use, particularly after prolonged activity, and is usually improved by rest. However, as the disease progresses, rest pain becomes more common. Joint pain is often difficult to localize and is frequently exacerbated by cold and damp weather. Early in the disease, patients feel stiffness, especially in the morning and after periods of inactivity, but measured loss of motion is minimal. In OA, periods of stiffness are typically less than 30 minutes, while RA patients can have prolonged periods of stiffness.

Loss of function results from a combination of pain, stiffness, deformity, contractures, muscle spasm, and muscle atrophy. Understanding the severity of actual disability is

Table 12-1

Helpful Hints

	OSTEOARTHRITIS	RHEUMATOID ARTHRITIS	REACTIVE/ CRYSTALLINE	INFECTION
Onset	Gradual	Gradual with recurrent acute flares	Acute, recurrent	Acute
Joint involvement	Often asymmetric, monoarticular	Symmetric, polyarticular	Usually monoarticular	Usually monoarticular
Systemic symptoms	None	With or without fever	May have fever, rash, diarrhea, urethritis, uveitis	Fever, chills
Age	Generally > 40 years	Onset generally 20 to 60 years	Any age	Any age
Other	History of repetitive use of joint	Family history	Medication use, family history	Tick exposure, sexual risk factors, other illness, IV drug use, travel outside country

paramount to properly treating the patient. In some cases, radiographs indicate severe disease, but the patient claims good function with minimal impact on personal, recreational, or vocational activities (Table 12-1).

EXAMINATION

To determine the overall impact of the arthritis, a comprehensive physical examination including the hand, wrist, elbow, and shoulder is necessary. A systematic approach to the examination includes inspection, palpation, assessing both active and passive range of motion, strength testing, neurovascular assessment, and tests specific to the joint of concern. Joint enlargement, redness, deformity, and tenderness are hallmarks of inflammation. Isolating points of tenderness helps the examiner reproduce the patient's symptoms and identify the source of pain.

Hand

The DIP joint is the most common joint of the hand afflicted by osteoarthritis (OA). Both pain and deformity are the primary concerns of the patient; however, the pain tends to be intermittent and often gradually improves, despite progressive deformity in some cases. Osteophyte formation involving the dorsal margin of the joint is the hallmark physical feature. The osteophytes produce visible and palpable enlargements termed *Heberden's nodes* (Table 12-2). In more advanced arthritis, the DIP joint can develop deformity in the form of a droop or lateral deviation. Occasionally, "mucous" cysts, which contain clear fluid, form over the joint, (see Table 12-2). The cyst may cause the overlying skin to thin, resulting in spontaneous rupture. Nail plate deformity distal to the cyst is also common due to pressure on the nail bed. The cysts can be quite painful, and patients often choose surgical excision.

Although less common, similar changes can occur in the PIP joints due to OA. The osteophytic enlargements are termed *Bouchard's nodes*. PIP joint stiffness is more disabling than DIP joint stiffness, and thus patients complain of decreased dexterity in addition to the pain. Stenosing flexor tenosynovitis (trigger finger) can sometimes mimic PIP arthritis. MCP joint OA is the least common site in the fingers, but there is predisposition in the index and long fingers, particularly in men. Pseudogout and hemochromatosis also affect the MCP joints, and thus a broader medical workup may be indicated. In some individuals with a strong family history, advanced OA can involve multiple joints in multiple digits, resulting in asymmetrical deformities that create a snake-like appearance of the fingers. When severe periarticular erosions and more obvious inflammation are present, the term *erosive osteoarthritis* is sometimes used.

The first CMC joint is the second-most common location of OA in the hand but is the most frequent cause of functional

Table 12-2

Methods for Examination

EXAM-INATION	TECHNIQUE	ILLUSTRATION	SIGNIFICANCE
Heberden node		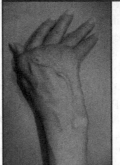	Osteoarthritis
Mucous cyst			Osteoarthritis
Grind test	Axial compression, flexion, extension, and circumduction of the first CMC joint		First CMC arthritis
Ulnar drift			Rheumatoid arthritis

(continued)

Table 12-2 (continued)

Methods for Examination

EXAM- INATION	TECHNIQUE	ILLUSTRATION	SIGNIFICANCE
Swan neck deformity		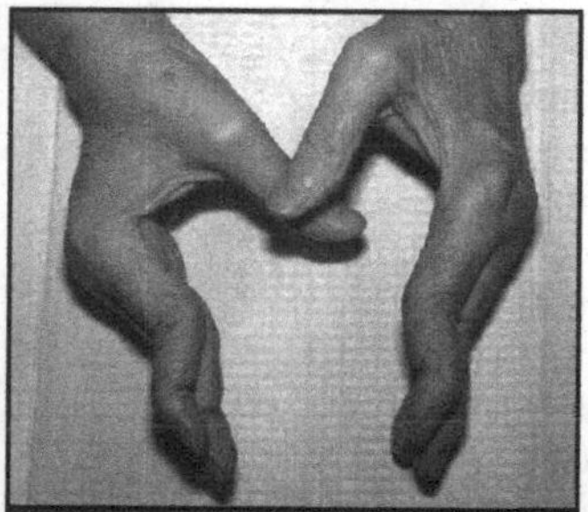	Rheumatoid arthritis
Boutonierre deformity		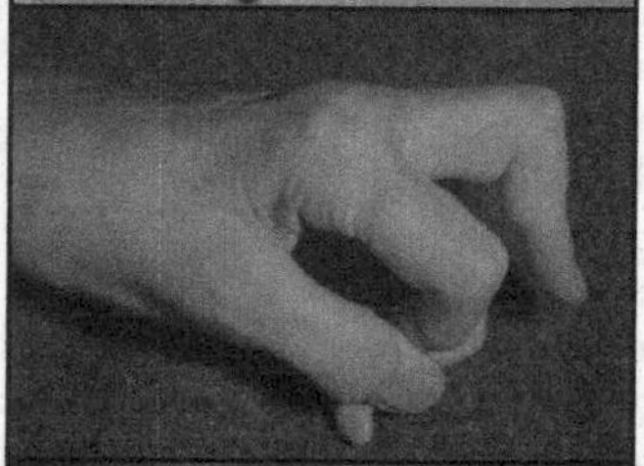	Rheumatoid arthritis
Rheumatoid nodules		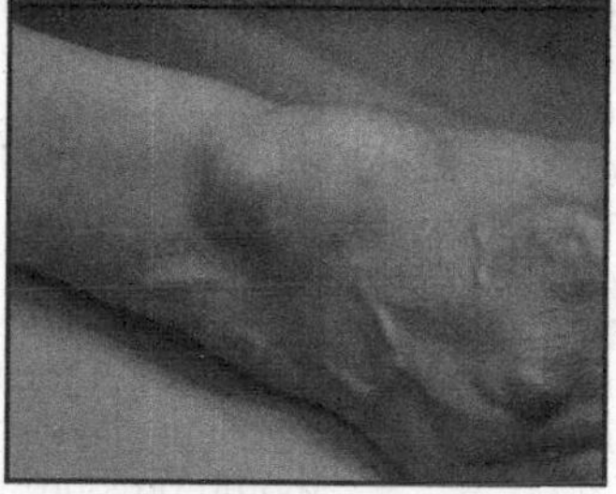	Rheumatoid arthritis
Piso-triquetral grind test	Grasp the pisiform between the index and thumb and displace it ulnar and radial to reproduce pain or crep-itus between the pisiform and trique-trum		Pisotriquetral osteoarthritis

(continued)

Table 12-2 (continued)

Methods for Examination

EXAMINATION	TECHNIQUE	ILLUSTRATION	SIGNIFICANCE
Scaphoid shift test	Slightly pronate the forearm, place the thumb on the palmar prominence of the scaphoid with the fingers wrapped around the distal radius, push on the scaphoid with counterpressure from the fingers, and then, starting in ulnar deviation and slight extension, bring the wrist radial and into flexion with constant thumb pressure on the scaphoid	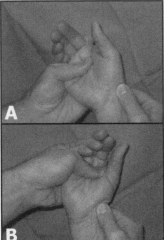 (A) Start in ulnar deviation and extension with the thumb on the palmar prominence of the scaphoid with the fingers wrapped around the distal radius, pushing on the scaphoid with counter-pressure from the fingers. (B) Bring the wrist radial and into flexion with constant thumb pressure.	Scaphoid instability/Radio-scaphoid OA
Hourglass at dorsal wrist		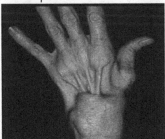	Wrist extensor compartment synovitis in RA

(continued)

Table 12-2 (continued)

Methods for Examination

EXAM- INATION	TECHNIQUE	ILLUSTRATION	SIGNIFICANCE
Shear or ballotte- ment test	Stabilize the lunate between the thumb and index finger of one hand while manu- ally shearing the triquetrum against the lunate articu- lar surface in a dorso-palmar direction with the thumb and index finger of the other hand		Lunotriquetral OA
Anterior and ulnar wrist sublux- ation		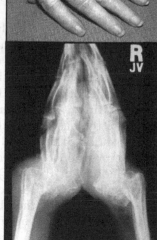	Rheumatoid arthritis

(continued)

Table 12-2 (continued)

Methods for Examination

Exam-ination	Technique	Illustration	Significance
Wrist instabil-ity	Grasp the lower forearm firmly in one hand and the hand and the carpus in the other with alternate dorsal and palmar movement of the hand to reveal instability		Rheumatoid arthritis
Piano key sign	Depress the ulnar head and then release; the ulnar head returns to its dorsal position		Rheumatoid arthritis

disability due to the importance of the thumb. Other causes of pain in this region of the hand must also be considered, including carpal tunnel syndrome, de Quervain's disease, stenosing flexor tenosynovitis, and wrist arthritis. On physical examination, there is tenderness over the joint line, which can usually be palpated directly, and often a squared appearance on the radial side of the base of the thumb ("shoulder sign") due to joint subluxation. The "grind test" is performed by applying axial compression combined with passive circumduction (circular motion of the joint), which produces pain and crepitance (see Table 12-2). A secondary hyperextension and abduction deformity of the thumb MCP joint is common, as the patient attempts to make up for the loss of first CMC abduction and overall motion.

The rheumatoid hand is characterized by certain patterns of deformities that have descriptive terms, including "ulnar drift," "swan neck," and "boutonniere" (see Table 12-2).[3] These deformities are caused by a combination of articular erosions and soft-tissue laxity. Ulnar drift refers to ulnar deviation of the fingers at the MCP joints, which usually develops gradually and involves all fingers of that hand. As the deformity becomes more severe, palmar-ward subluxation of the joints occurs, leading to greater loss of motion and dexterity. Swan neck refers to hyperextension at the PIP and flexion at the DIP joint, which can be a flexible or fixed deformity that reduces grip strength. Boutonniere deformity describes flexion at the PIP joint and hyperextension at the DIP joint, which also can be flexible or fixed but causes less loss of function. The thumb can develop similar changes, but a boutonniere deformity is the most common. As opposed to OA patients, patients with RA usually have a more symmetrical distribution of joint involvement; however, the severity of deformity can substantially vary. Joints with severe erosions become flail and digits shorten. With traction, folds in the redundant skin telescope out, hence the term *opera glass hand* applied to a hand with severe disease.

Rheumatoid nodules are a common feature of the disease and are typically found over the extensor surfaces of the hands and arms (see Table 12-2). They are firm and rubbery and can become very large. In addition to the 3 common deformities already listed, other common hand deformities in RA include palmar subluxation of the MCP joints, Z-deformity of the thumb, lateral dislocation of the IP joints, and misalignment of the digits, suggestive of tendon rupture.

Wrist

Wrist OA is relatively common but frequently tolerated and responsive to routine medications, rest, and modification of activities. However, some patients develop substantial swelling and pain. Joint line tenderness is particularly helpful to assess the location of the arthritis, but confirmation with radiographs is often necessary to determine its true location. The most common pattern of wrist arthritis is called the scapholunate advanced collapse (SLAC) wrist, which begins at the articulation between the radius and scaphoid and progresses in a specific pattern to involve scaphocapitate and capitolunate articulations arthritis followed by generalized wrist arthritis. This pattern is thought to be initiated by or at least accelerated by a tear of the scapholunate interosseous ligament. A variation of the SLAC wrist is the scaphoid nonunion advanced collapse (SNAC) wrist, which implies a longstanding nonunion of the scaphoid that causes malalignment of the carpus that induces degenerative changes. Clinical examination will reveal swelling and tenderness in the "anatomic snuff box," which is the normal depression over the dorsal radial aspect of the wrist and anatomically lies over the scaphoid between the first and second dorsal extensor tendon compartments. This normal depression becomes reversed to become a prominence due to swelling. Unless wrist stiffness has developed, the scaphoid shift test is positive. This is begun by slightly pronating the forearm, placing the thumb on the palmar prominence of the distal scaphoid, and wrapping the fingers around the distal radius. While applying pressure on the scaphoid with the thumb and counter-pressure with the fingers, the wrist is moved from ulnar deviation and slight extension into radial deviation and slight flexion (see Table 12-2).[4] In radioscaphoid arthritis, this maneuver usually results in pain; relative hypermobility of the scaphoid; and sometimes crepitance, clicking, or a "clunk." Comparison should be made with the opposite wrist.

The second-most common site of wrist OA is at the scaphotrapezialtrapezoid joint. Examination will reveal swelling and fullness slightly more distal than radioscaphoid arthritis. There may also be swelling on the volar radial aspect of the wrist. The palmar scaphoid and the distal flexor carpi radialis tendon are tender. Radial ulnar deviation of the wrist typically causes pain because the joint undergoes the greatest motion during this movement.

The ulnar side of the wrist requires an especially careful exam, as several important structures are located in this small anatomic area. Thus, in palpating for tenderness, it is best to use a single fingertip to better isolate potential pathological sites. Because the DRUJ, ulnocarpal joint, lunotriquetral joint, and proximal radioulnar joint are closely linked anatomically and functionally, an examination of all joints and structures is essential to ensure that symptoms are being attributed to the correct source. Instability due to ligament injury or degeneration due to OA or post-traumatic arthritis are the most common problems.[5] The DRUJ, wrist, and forearm are examined both volarly and dorsally and are compared to the other side because there is high variability in the normal anatomy and stability in this region. Decreased motion and crepitus during pronation and supination are signs of DRUJ arthritis, which may be accentuated by manually compressing the joint. The lunotriquetral (LT) joint is identified just distal and radial to the ulnar styloid. It can be stressed using the shear or ballottement test. In this test, the examiner stabilizes the lunate between the thumb and index finger of one hand while manipulating the triquetrum against the lunate in a dorso-palmar direction with the thumb and index finger of the other hand. In pisotriquetral arthritis, pressing and manipulating the pisiform will elicit pain and crepitus. This can be accentuated by having the patient clench the fingers.

In the rheumatoid patient, wrist swelling can be due to tenosynovitis involving either the flexor or extensor tendons surrounding the wrist or from synovitis of the wrist joint itself. In many cases, there is a combination of these conditions, which can make it difficult to determine the primary source of swelling. Furthermore, within the wrist joint, there are 3 compartments that can become involved individually or in combination: the radiocarpal joint, the midcarpal joint, and the radioulnar joint. Flexor tenosynovitis may cause distal forearm swelling that can extend into the palm. It is associated with crepitus during active finger motion and may be first diagnosed by causing carpal tunnel syndrome. Tenosynovitis of the extensor tendon is characterized by an hour-glass appearance, with the narrowing due to containment by the extensor retinaculum (see Table 12-2). Extensor tenosynovitis can cause tendon subluxations and ruptures, resulting in loss of finger or wrist motion and deformities of the joints (see Table 12-2). Because extensor and flexor tenosynovitis can be relatively painless, sudden loss of active motion can be the presenting complaint. Progressive wrist arthritis results in the classic rheumatoid wrist deformity manifested by radial deviation, ulnar translocation, supination, and eventually volar subluxation. Osteophytes on the scaphoid may cause erosive ruptures of the flexor pollicis longus tendons. The distal radioulnar joint is typically involved early, which creates instability and dorsal subluxation of the ulna and adds to the apparent deformity (see Table 12-2). The prominent ulna may cause attrition ruptures of the small and ring finger extensor tendons (see Table 12-2).

PATHOANATOMY

Osteoarthritis

The pathophysiology of OA is an area of increasing research because of its huge impact on quality of life and economics. It is a progressive deterioration of articular cartilage characterized by fissuring and focal erosions accompanied by an attempted repair and remodeling response.[6] The overall health of articular cartilage relies on the chondrocytes, which synthesize collagens, proteoglycans, and proteinases. When the chondrocytes fail to maintain the balance between synthesis and degradation of the extracellular matrix, the continuity, resistance, and elasticity of the cartilage is reduced.[7] In addition, with aging, chondrocytes shift from production of Type II collagen to production of Types I and III collagens and to synthesis of shorter proteoglycans.[8]

Rheumatoid Arthritis

RA is caused by an aberrant immune response in a genetically predisposed individual, leading to chronic progressive synovial inflammation and subsequent joint destruction.[9] The genetic basis is complex, and the precipitating factors have not been identified. It remains a matter of debate whether the disease is triggered by an infectious agent, a breach in tolerance leading to autoimmunity, or an accumulation of events that occur with age. The synovial membrane undergoes dramatic changes including hyperplasia, an influx of inflammatory cells, and release of enzymes into the synovial fluid, resulting in destruction of articular cartilage, ligaments, tendons, and bone. Bone erosions occur at the junction of bone and cartilage and are frequently associated with a hypertrophic synovial-like extension called a pannus. The pannus causes rapid joint injury through production of proteinases that degrade collagen and proteoglycans. Macrophages are induced to

Table 12-3

Imaging

	OA	RA	REACTIVE/ CRYSTALLINE	INFECTION
Radiographs	Asymmetric joint space narrowing, osteophytes, sclerosis, cysts	Erosions, osteopenia, effusion, soft tissue swelling, deformity, and malalignment	Erosions, possible crystal deposition	Effusion, soft tissue swelling

become osteoclasts, resulting in further erosion. Ligaments become attenuated by chronic swelling and the inflammatory response, which leads to joint deformities.

IMAGING

Hand

Three views of the hand (posterior-anterior [PA], lateral, and oblique) are typically obtained to evaluate joint disease in the hand. When a specific digit is involved, isolating that digit in the radiographs is helpful to avoid obscuring detail by overlap with other digits. Joint space loss, erosions, osteophytes, and malalignment are the key findings of OA (Table 12-3). If first CMC arthritis is suspected, a PA, lateral, or view or Bett view will best image the joint (Figure 12-1) and will demonstrate if trapezioscaphoid arthritis is also present. In general, no advanced imaging is necessary for the evaluation of hand arthritis.

Wrist

PA, lateral, and oblique views of the wrist are the usual views in an initial evaluation for suspected wrist arthritis.

Figure 12-1. Eaton view. All articulations of the trapezium are projected without overlap from the surrounding bones.

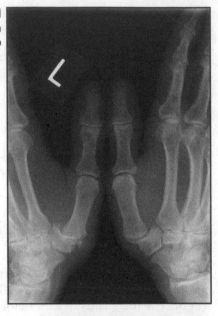

Figure 12-2. Complete loss of radioscaphoid joint space with widening of the scapholunate interval and preserved joint space at the lunate fossa consistent with scapholunate advance collapse (SLAC) wrist.

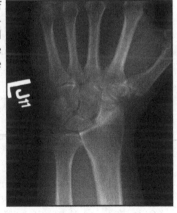

The characteristic pattern of degeneration is seen in SLAC and scaphoid nonunion advanced collapse (SNAC) wrists (Figure 12-2). In osteonecrosis of the lunate (Kienböck's disease), there is increased density or sclerosis and possibly collapse of the lunate, resulting in progressive malalignment of the carpus and arthritis. Early Kienböck's disease can be difficult to assess in standard radiographs, but MRI can usually confirm the diagnosis. Distal radioulnar joint arthritis usually begins with osteophyte formation on the proximal margin of the ulnar head and progresses to have the typical findings of OA with sclerosis and loss of joint space. *Ulnar impaction syndrome* is a term applied to degeneration of the ulnocarpal joint and is caused by repetitive excessive loading between the ulnar head and carpus, resulting in sclerosis and cystic changes in the dome of the ulna, lunate, and triquetrum. Ulnar-positive variance, which is a description indicating the ulna is longer than the radius at the level of the wrist, is a predisposition to ulnar impaction syndrome because it may increase the relative load across the wrist at this site. The triangular fibrocartilage (TFC), which forms a cushion within this articulation, also undergoes degenerative wear. Unless it is involved with chondrocalcinosis, indicated by trace calcifications, the degenerative changes in the TFC can only be imaged by either MRI or arthroscopy.

Elbow

Two views are often not sufficient to evaluate elbow arthritis; oblique views better demonstrate the osteophytes and loose bodies associated with elbow OA. The medial oblique view shows the trochlea, olecranon, and coronoid, while the lateral oblique view shows the medial epicondyle, radioulnar joint, and coronoid tubercle. An axial view with the patient's elbow flexed 110 degrees, the forearm on the cassette, and the beam directed perpendicular will better show the epicondyles, ulnar sulcus, and radiocapitellar and ulnotrochlear articulations. In stiff elbows, a CT scan may be the most practical method to adequately visualize the joint (see Table 12-3).

TREATMENT

The initial treatment of arthritis, whether of the hand, wrist, or elbow, is nearly always nonsurgical. Activity modification, splinting, anti-inflammatory medications, and periodic intra-articular steroid injections can benefit most patients at least initially and may lead to avoidance or delay of surgical intervention. Surgical management usually considered only if these measures fail. The medical management of RA using disease-modifying anti-rheumatic drugs (DMARDs) has resulted in a marked decrease in the incidence of the severe deformities seen in rheumatoid patients and a drastic reduction in the need for surgical management.

Hand

Surgical interventions for hand OA include removal of symptomatic cysts, joint débridement in select cases, arthrodesis, and arthroplasty. Thumb CMC arthritis is occasionally managed in selected patients with mild arthritis by joint preservation operations, including volar ligament reconstruction, metacarpal extension osteotomy, or arthroscopic debridement. Once degenerative changes are advanced, arthrodesis or resectional arthroplasty with or without ligament reconstruction and tendon interposition (LRTI) are the preferred surgical options.[10] Implant arthroplasty has yet to achieve predictably good outcomes for thumb CMC arthritis, but in selected patients with otherwise good joint alignment and bone and soft-tissue quality, an implant arthroplasty may provide more rapid pain relief and better function.

Surgical excision is the preferred treatment for a persistent and painful mucous cyst due to DIP joint OA, particularly if it is draining or causing nail deformity. The excision includes removal of the offending osteophyte to reduce the risk of recurrence. When the pain is associated with deformity and stiffness, fusion of the joint is the best option.

Although PIP OA is best treated by arthrodesis because of the high demands on the joint, the lost motion substantially reduces finger function, especially in the small and ring fingers. Thus, in selected patients with PIP arthritis but otherwise good joint alignment, an implant can be considered.

The most common surgical procedures for RA of the hand include tenosynovectomy, soft-tissue rebalancing, tendon transfers, arthrodesis, and silicone implant arthroplasty (primarily reserved for the MP joints). Although procedures that preserve motion will improve joint alignment initially, recurrence of deformity is common. Thus, these procedures are not typically performed early in the disease. Conversely, in patients with unremitting disease and advancing deformity, early surgical treatment is best in order to preserve overall hand function.

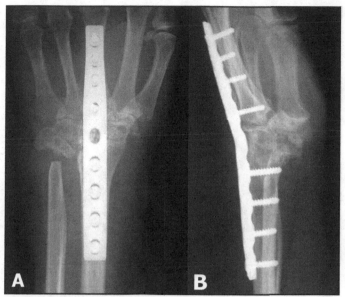

Figure 12-3. Wrist fusion radiographs: (A) AP and (B) lateral.

Wrist

Surgical options for advanced wrist OA (SLAC, SNAC wrist) include radial styloid excision, proximal row carpectomy, scaphoid excision with intercarpal arthrodesis (capitohamate-lunotriquetral arthrodesis), and implant arthroplasty (Figures 12-3 and 12-4).[11,12] Each of these procedures can be very effective, with the choice individualized to the patient's arthritis severity, age, and activity demands. For DRUJ arthritis, ulnar shortening (for early stage OA), resection arthroplasty (Darrach procedure, hemiresection-interposition arthroplasty), arthrodesis (Sauvé-Kapandji procedure), and distal ulnar head implant arthroplasty are options (Figure 12-5).[5] Again, the chosen procedure depends on a combination of patient needs and the joint condition.

Surgical treatment of the wrist in RA is highly dependent on the severity of the deformity. If the pain is tolerable and the wrist is adequately aligned with minimal shortening, then surgery should be delayed. However, because the wrist is the foundation for hand function, severe deformity should be

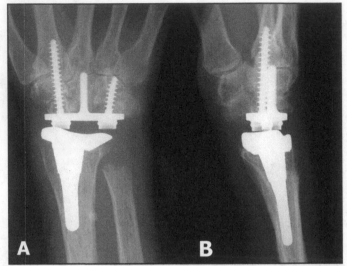

Figure 12-4. Wrist arthroplasty radiographs: (A) AP and (B) lateral.

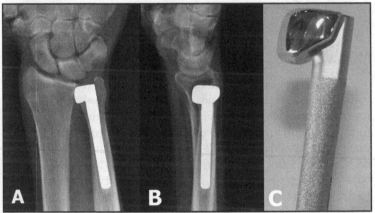

Figure 12-5. Partial ulnar head arthroplasty, (A) AP and (B) lateral, and (C) photograph of the implant.

avoided. Radiolunate arthrodesis is indicated for early arthritis with progressive deformity, while complete arthrodesis is the standard for most patients. Total wrist arthroplasty is considered for patients with bilateral disease and adequate tissue quality. For advanced DRUJ arthritis, most RA patients are treated by a resection of the distal ulna (Darrach procedure).

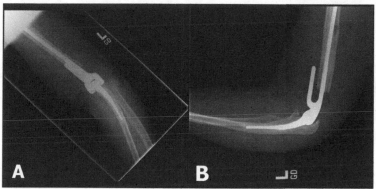

Figure 12-6. Total elbow arthroplasty, AP and lateral.

Elbow

Surgical options for elbow OA and post-traumatic arthritis include open or arthroscopic joint debridement with removal of impinging osteophytes and loose bodies. Ulnohumeral arthroplasty, often called the "OK procedure" because it was described by Outerbridge and popularized by Kashiwagi, is a technique that decompresses the posterior elbow compartment using a large trephine via a posterior approach. By removing this hypertrophic bone, there is increased space posteriorly for elbow extension. The large hole through the olecranon fossa provides access to the anterior compartment for removal of loose bodies, resection of osteophytes, and removal of the prominent coronoid tip. In patients with greater involvement of the radiocapitellar joint, resection of the radial head with or without implant replacement is a very successful procedure. Total elbow arthroplasty is rarely indicated for OA of the elbow because these patients are usually younger, more active, and at high risk for implant failure.[13]

For early or moderate RA of the elbow, open or arthroscopic synovectomy may provide pain relief and may potentially prolong the life of the joint. Synovectomy is often combined with radial head excision. Total elbow arthroplasty is a reasonable alternative for those with more advanced disease (Figure 12-6).[14]

CONCLUSION

Arthritis of the hand, wrist, and elbow is common and is usually managed conservatively in its early stages. For severe arthritis, surgical treatment is effective for specific joints but must be individualized to the patient to provide a predictable outcome. Rheumatoid patients have special considerations and often different treatment alternatives than those with OA or post-traumatic arthritis.

REFERENCES

1. Sharma L. Epidemiology of osteoarthritis. In: Moskowitz RW, Howell DS, Altman RD, Buckwalter JA, Goldberg VM, eds. *Osteoarthritis, Third edition: Diagnosis and Medical/Surgical Management.* Philadelphia: WB Saunders Company; 2001:3-27.
2. Chaisson CE, Zhang Y, McAlindon TE. Radiographic hand osteoarthritis: incidence, patterns, and influence of pre-existing disease in a population based sample. *J Rheumatol.* 1997;24:1337-1343.
3. Smith P. Rheumatoid arthritis, its variants, and osteoarthritis. In: Smith P. Lister. *The Hand: Diagnosis and Indications, Fourth Edition.* London, UK: Harcourt Publishers; 2002:331-398.
4. Cooney WP, Bishop AT, Linscheid RL. Physical examination of the wrist. In: Cooney WP, Linscheid RL, Dobyns JH, eds. *The Wrist: Diagnosis and Operative Treatment.* St. Louis, MO: Mosby; 1998:236-261.
5. Adams BD. Distal radioulnar joint instability. In: Green DP, Hotchkiss RN, Pederson, WC, Wolfe SW, eds. *Green's Operative Hand Surgery, Fifth Edition.* Philadelphia, PA: Elsevier Churchill Livingstone; 2005:605-644.
6. Mankin HJ, Mow VC, Buckwalter JA. Articular cartilage repair and osteoarthritis. In: Buckwalter JA, Einhorn TA, Simon SR, eds. *Orthopaedic Basic Science: Biology and Biomechanics of the Musculoskeletal System, Second Edition.* Rosemont, IL: American Academy of Orthopaedic Surgeons; 2000:471-488.
7. Berenbaum F. Osteoarthritis: Epidemiology, pathology, and pathogenesis. In: Klippel JH, ed. *Primer on the Rheumatic Diseases.* Atlanta, GA: Arthritis Foundation; 2001:285-289.
8. Goldring MB. The role of the chondrocyte in osteoarthritis. *Arthritis Rheum.* 2000;43:1916-1926.
9. Boumpas DT, Illei GG, Tassiulas IO. Rheumatoid arthritis. In: Klippel JH, ed. *Primer on the Rheumatic Diseases.* Atlanta, GA: Arthritis Foundation; 2001:209-232.
10. Van Heest AE, Kallemeier P. Thumb carpal metacarpal arthritis. *J Am Acad Orthop Surg.* 2008;16(3):140-151.
11. Wyrick JD. Proximal row carpectomy and intercarpal arthrodesis for the management of wrist arthritis. *J Am Acad Orthop Surg.* 2003;11:277-281.

12. Cooney WP, DeBartolo T, Wood, MB. Post-traumatic arthritis of the wrist. In: Cooney WP, Linscheid RL, Dobyns JH, eds. *The Wrist: Diagnosis and Operative Treatment.* St. Louis, MO: Mosby; 1998:588-631.
13. Gramstad GD, Galatz LM. Management of elbow osteoarthritis. *J Bone Joint Surg Am.* 2006;88:421-430.
14. Kauffman JI, Chen AL, Stuchin S, Di Cesare PE. Surgical management of the rheumatoid elbow. *J Am Acad Orthop Surg.* 2003;11:100-108.

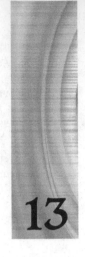

13

Examination of Elbow, Wrist, and Hand Fractures

David Ring, MD, PhD

Introduction

There are several aspects of the physical examination for fractures that are common to all anatomical areas in the arm. Inspection for wounds, swelling, ecchymosis, and deformity is the first step. If there is no gross deformity or instability of the limb and the patient is reasonably comfortable, I ask the patient to demonstrate range of motion next. I consider this part of the "inspection" of a limb. I think it provides very useful information about the location and severity of the injury as

Culp RW, Jacoby SM. *Musculoskeletal Examination of the Elbow, Wrist, and Hand: Making the Complex Simple* (pp. 274-290). © 2012 Taylor & Francis Group.

well as about the patient's cognitive and emotional reaction to the injury (based on how much the pain is unsettling to him or her in comparison to what we would expect for that particular injury). It also tells me the status of the musculotendinous units. Fractures are either stable or unstable, so the concern that attempting range of motion prior to radiographic definition of the injury has little merit.

Next, I palpate the arm systematically, leaving the likely focus of the injury for last. During palpation, I look for tenderness, both in the patient's report and in his or her facial expression or retraction of the limb. The degree of retraction can also give me an idea of how unsettling the injury has been for the patient. Because trauma should cause a discrete area of tenderness, more diffuse tenderness can also indicate uneasiness. I systematically examine all areas of potential concern. For instance, I always evaluate the scaphoid because I do not want to overlook an occult or subtle fracture and the distal radius, because it is so commonly fractured.

When I palpate the likely area of fracture, I evaluate deformity by assessing anatomical landmarks for normal relationships. I also assess for crepitation, particularly with joint motion. In the obtunded patient, crepitation can be the only evidence of fracture rather than contusion or sprain. I do not test stability until I have seen the radiographs.

Finally, I do a neurovascular examination. I check light touch sensation, move on to static two-point discrimination if there are issues, and use simple pin prick when the arm is mangled enough that two-point discrimination will be tricky or if there is altered consciousness and limited patient cooperation. For the motor exam, I check hyperextension of the thumb IP joint and wrist extension (radial nerve), first dorsal interosseous and small finger flexor pollicis longus (ulnar nerve), and palmar abduction of the thumb and the index flexor pollicis longus (median nerve) and do more if I find abnormalities or inconsistencies.

HISTORY

Details about the patient, including age, gender, health, activity level, etc, will affect interpretation of the injury as well as management, as will knowledge of the injury mechanism, including energy, associated injuries, contamination, etc. The timing and prior treatment are also important. Nerve dysfunction and compartment syndrome are suspected based on the patient's reports of numbness or disproportionate pain, respectively. It is also important to understand the patient's goals, preferences, and risk tolerance.

ELBOW DISLOCATIONS AND FRACTURES

Elbow Dislocation

After attempted reduction of an elbow dislocation, palpation can confirm realignment prior to radiographs. There is a triangle formed by the medial and lateral epicondyles and the point of the olecranon process. This triangle should form a plane that is parallel to the axis of the humerus. If the elbow dislocated or subluxated, these relationships will be disrupted.[1]

Stability is tested by having the patient straighten his or her elbow to see if it dislocates again. This can only be tested if the patient is sufficiently conscious to participate, but sufficiently anesthetized to put the elbow back in again if it comes out. Varus and valgus stability can be tested, but it will not affect management; we expect complete capsuloligamentous injury in the vast majority of elbow dislocations, so establishing that by testing varus and valgus will not add information. On the other hand, if there is stability to valgus stress, it may be that you are treating a patient with the unusual elbow that has dislocated with the anterior band of the MCL at least partially spared[2] (Table 13-1).

Postoperative radiographs should demonstrate concentric reduction. If there is a sag of the elbow—the so-called "drop sign"—teach the patient active flexion exercises from 90 degrees to the maximum tolerated and have the lateral radiograph repeated, but without the usual abduction of the shoulder (which placed a posterolateral rotatory stress on the elbow and caused it to subluxate) (Figure 13-1).[3] If a lateral radiograph made with active flexion and no varus or valgus stress shows concentric reduction, then the patient can be instructed to avoid shoulder abduction and perform frequent

Table 13-1

Helpful Hints

CONDITION

Stability after elbow dislocation	Test varus and valgus instability if you're curious (sometimes the anterior band of the MCL is intact), but it won't change management.	We expect everything to be torn, so the only "instability" we are interested in is if the elbow redislocates as it approaches extension.
Slight sag in the elbow after reduction	This is called the "drop sign" (see Figure 13-1) and is analogous to pseudosubluxation in the shoulder.	Have the patient work on active flexion exercises and avoid varus stress (shoulder abduction). Take the lateral x-ray with the shoulder forward flexed and in front of the body rather than abducted and placed on a table.
Isolated radial head fractures	While we worry about the fracture blocking forearm rotation, this rarely occurs. The elbow effusion hurts a great deal, so the exam may be incomplete initially.	There's no harm in waiting up to 1 week, at which time the patient will be much more comfortable. Alternatively one can aspirate the hemarthrosis and put in some anesthetic to make it easier to evaluate forearm rotation. (see Table 13-1).
Radial head excision	It's unusual to treat a radial head fracture with simple excision. If it seems like a reasonable option, make sure there is no forearm instability with the push-pull maneuver and that the MCL and LCL are intact using valgus stress and the elbow pivot shift.	The push-pull test for interosseous ligament injury is just grabbing the wrist and placing axial load and traction looking for substantial translation—the radial neck will collide with the capitellum. It is not a subtle finding.

(continued)

Table 13-1 (continued)

Helpful Hints

CONDITION

Coronoid fractures	Small, isolated coronoid fractures often involve the anteromedial facet and have an associated LCL injury.	Apply a varus stress and take an x-ray to see if there is subluxation of the elbow indicating LCL injury. If the elbow sits in a subluxated position, surgery is preferable.
DRUJ instability	There is no consensus on the definition and objective measurement of DRUJ instability.	The key is to assess the patient's uninjured wrist. Use the piano key sign (see Table 13-1). After repair of any fractures, if the DRUJ stability is comparable to the opposite side, nothing more needs to be done.
Scaphoid fractures	There is no consensus reference standard for a true fracture among suspected fractures. The diagnosis of a suspected scaphoid fracture is commonly made in the United States where the prevalence of true fractures among suspected fractures is less than 10% compared to 15% to 20% in Europe.	The scaphoid can be palpated for tenderness both in the anatomic snuffbox (see Table 13-1) as well as over the distal pole (see Figure 13-5B). If the patient is diffusely tender DO NOT document these signs as positive, just document the diffuse tenderness and wait 1 or 2 weeks for things to settle prior to re-examining.

active elbow flexion exercises, and this should allow the ligaments to heal with the elbow in concentric alignment.[4] Patients may not be capable of doing all of this immediately after elbow dislocation, and it is reasonable to do this a few days to a week later in the office, splinting the patient initially. This same approach—adding the dynamic component of elbow stability—can also be useful after operative treatment of elbow instability.

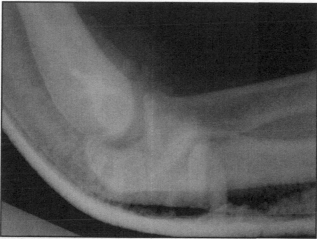

Figure 13-1. Lateral radiograph 5 days after reduction of an elbow dislocation shows a "drop sign" or pseudosubluxation of the elbow. This resolved with active exercises and avoidance of shoulder abduction (varus stress) for 3 to 4 weeks.

Radial Head Fractures

A suspected occult radial head fracture can be confirmed by a point of maximal tenderness over the radial head. For displaced radial head fractures being considered for operative treatment, substantial crepitation over the radial head with forearm rotation or a true block to motion (not just reluctance to move due to pain) might increase the appeal of operative treatment. When the lack of forearm rotation seems like it may be due to pain, one can either re-examine the patient in a few days when the pain has calmed or aspirate the blood from the joint with or without injection of a local anesthetic. The center of the triangle formed by the lateral epicondyle, the point of the olecranon, and the radial head is the so-called "soft-spot" of the elbow, which represents the best place to aspirate or inject the elbow joint (Table 13-2).

During operative treatment of a fracture of the radial head, one should test for associated ligament injuries. After induction of anesthesia and before preparation and draping of the joint, stability can be tested by applying a valgus stress with the elbow in 20 degrees of flexion under the image intensifier.

Table 13-2

Methods for Examination

MANEUVER	DESCRIPTION	ILLUSTRATION
Aspiration or injection of the elbow joint	There is a soft spot between the radial head, the lateral epicondyle, and the olecranon below.	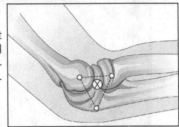

The so-called "soft spot" between the lateral epicondyle, radial head, and olecranon is a useful area for aspiration or injection of the elbow joint.

| Test for posterolateral rotatory instability (insufficiency of the lateral collateral ligament complex) of the elbow | Try to push the radial head behind the capitellum with axial load, forceful maximum supination and extension, and valgus stress. 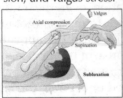 | Look for a dimple and a clunk with reduction as the elbow is flexed. 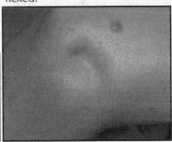 |

The so-called "pivot shift" of the elbow elicited as a clunk when moving from extension, valgus, axial, and supination stress to flexion.

(continued)

Table 13-2 (continued)

Methods for Examination

MANEUVER	DESCRIPTION	ILLUSTRATION
DRUJ instability	Stablize the radius. Grab the ulna in your hand and try to shift it anterior and posterior with respect to the radius. Compare to the opposite side	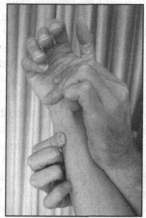

Instability of the distal ulna is tested by grasping the hand and radius and the distal ulna separately and maximally subluxating the ulna dorsal and volar. This should be compared to the other side.

Scaphoid fractures	The scaphoid can be palpated in the so-called "snuffbox" between the EPL and the EPB/APL tendons on the radial side of the wrist. The distal pole of the scaphoid can be palpated at the transverse wrist creases.	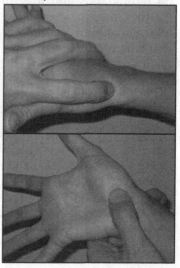

WRIST FRACTURES

Scaphoid Fracture

The scaphoid can be palpated not only in the anatomical snuffbox (see Table 13-2), but also over the distal pole of the scaphoid (prominent on the volar aspect of the wrist and hand, just distal to the transverse wrist creases) (see Table 13-2). Tenderness with axial compression of the thumb is also a useful sign of possible scaphoid fracture.[11] Any patient with tenderness in these areas after a fall onto the hand should be suspected of having an occult scaphoid fracture if there is neither a scaphoid fracture, nor another source for the tenderness seen on radiographs. Patients with intra-articular fractures will usually have diminished active wrist motion.

Triage of suspected scaphoid fractures has several approaches, and it is not clear which is best.[12] One or 2 weeks of rest and recovery can make the examination more reliable, and new radiographs can show the fracture. If after this interval the examination is still concerning and the radiographs (including scaphoid-specific views) are normal, then CT, magnetic resonance, or bone scan can be considered.

Diagnosis of scaphoid fracture displacement can be difficult on radiographs and may merit CT scanning.[12] A displaced fracture may be associated with some degree of ligament injury (a minor perilunate injury), although it is not clear that this merits any specific investigation or operative treatment—alignment and fixation of the scaphoid fracture seem sufficient.

Distal Radius Fractures

Displaced fractures of the distal radius are usually obvious. The median nerve should be evaluated prior to and after manipulative reduction and at all subsequent follow-up evaluations. Patients with high-energy fractures or widely displaced fractures should be advised of the possibility of acute carpal tunnel syndrome and even forearm compartment syndrome, and should be given contact information should numbness or extreme pain with finger motion begin to develop.

Substantial opening on the medial side indicates a medial collateral ligament (MCL) complex injury. The MCL injury does not need specific treatment as long as the radial head fracture is either repaired or replaced with a prosthesis.

The lateral collateral ligament is evaluated by testing varus stress with the elbow in 20 degrees of flexion, but also by testing for subluxation or dislocation with posterolateral rotatory instability. The latter is done by externally rotating the humerus over the head in order to lock the humerus and then applying an axial load, valgus stress, and forceful maximal supination to the radial head (see Table 13-2).[5] If you think of trying to force the radial head behind the capitellum, this is easier to remember. When operating on the radial head, always check the origin of the lateral collateral ligament from the lateral epicondyle. If this is avulsed, there was an elbow dislocation or near dislocation. The ligament injury can greatly facilitate exposure and should be repaired with suture anchors or drill holes through bone upon closure.

The interosseous ligament and the triangular fibrocartilage complex (TFCC) are tested using the so-called radius-pull test.[6] This can be done either after radial head excision or prior to incision by applying longitudinal axial compression and distraction and seeing how far the radius translates at the elbow and at the wrist. In the presence of a true acute Essex-Lopresti lesion (complete longitudinal instability of the forearm due to injury of the interosseous ligament and the TFCC), this test is not subtle. You should be able to hit the radial neck against the capitellum with the radial head excised. When to worry about lesser amounts of translation is unclear. More than 6 mm is felt to indicate an Essex-Lopresti lesion based on serial cutting studies in cadaver arm studies.[6]

Coronoid Fractures

Imaging of coronoid fractures with 2- and 3-dimensional reconstructions of computed tomography (CT) scans can give substantial information about the injury pattern, which will indicate the other structures likely to be injured.[7,8] For instance, a small transverse tip fracture of the coronoid is typical of posterolateral rotatory instability and is likely to be associated with injury to both collateral ligaments and the radial head. Fracture of the anteromedial facet of the coronoid is likely to be associated with either avulsion of the lateral col-lateral ligament origin or an olecranon fracture. Both collateral ligaments are likely injured if there was a complete elbow dislocation in association with a small anteromedial coronoid fracture. If there is subluxation of the trochlear anteriorly from the trochlear notch on the medial side, operative treatment is advisable, whereas concentric reduction can sometimes be managed nonoperatively with avoidance of varus stress and active flexion exercises. Large, basilar coronoid fractures are usually associated with olecranon fracture-dislocations.

It can be useful to look for these associated injuries using image intensification with or without anesthesia. Assessment of posterolateral rotatory instability (PLRI) was discussed above. When there is an isolated anteromedial coronoid frac-ture, varus stress is tested, and opening of the radiocapitellar joint is sought on the image intensifier.

Distal Humerus Fracture

Apparent capitellum fractures should be assessed with 3-dimensional CT reconstructions with the radius and the ulna subtracted.[9] In many cases, additional fractures, some of which are impacted and stable, will be identified. Prior to preparing the arm, an examination under the image intensi-fier can disclose injury to the MCL. Again, this will not need specific treatment provided that radiocapitellar contact and concentric elbow instability can be restored. The lateral collat-eral ligament/lateral epicondyle (often fractured) is assessed upon operative exploration. Because most of these injuries are treated operatively and many are imaged with CT scans, physical examination for LCL injury is unnecessary.

One simple way to get a better idea of what is going on in columnar fractures is to obtain radiographs with the elbow under axial traction. Some patients are comfortable enough or already sedated or obtunded that this can be done in the emer-gency room; otherwise, this can be done prior to operative treatment under the image intensifier in the operating room. I get excellent information from CT scans, particularly 3-dimen-sional reconstructions with the radius and ulna removed, so I rarely use traction views.

The Ulnar Nerve

It is now well recognized that ulnar nerve dysfunction is very common after operative treatment of distal humerus fractures and occurs within a few years in a substantial percentage of patients with other types of elbow injury, such as fracture-dislocations.[10] I suspect that it is often overlooked by patients and surgeons. We should examine the ulnar nerve prior to surgery, after surgery, and at each stage of follow-up. During follow-up, one can add Tinel's sign (tap over the course of the ulnar nerve—which may have been transposed) and an elbow flexion test (30 seconds or greater of maximum elbow flexion looking for numbness in the small finger).

FOREARM FRACTURES

Diaphyseal forearm fractures are usually obvious due to pain, instability, and deformity. The proximal and distal radioulnar joints should be carefully evaluated both clinically and radiographically. A line up the middle of the radial shaft should bisect the capitellum on any radiographic view—although it can sometimes be difficult to tell where the capitellum is on very oblique radiographs. Radiographic evaluation of the distal radioulnar joint is more difficult. On a true lateral radiograph (determined by seeing the volar margin of the pisiform between the volar margin of the distal pole of the scaphoid and the volar margin of the capitate on a lateral radiograph), the ulna should be in line with the radius. In questionable cases, CT with the forearm in neutral rotation will be needed.

The stability of the opposite, uninjured distal radioulnar joint should be evaluated for comparison because laxity and the ability to subluxate the DRUJ have a wide range of normal. The radius and ulna are grasped, and one attempts to dislocate the ulnar head from the lesser sigmoid notch of the distal radius (see Table 13-2). Rotation of the forearm with pressure between the bones should not cause dislocation. This examination is usually not possible until after the forearm bones have been repaired in the operating room.

Figure 13-2. A displaced fracture of the distal radius was associated with an ulnar wound where the ulna tore through the skin as it dislocated.

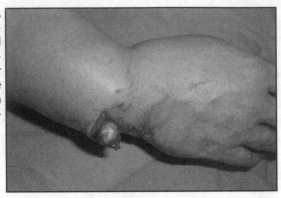

The radial styloid is a volar structure, and palpation can give an indication of alignment. After manipulative reduction, if the radial styloid is in a volar position, then the palmar tilt is likely restored.

For minimally displaced or nondisplaced fractures of the distal radius that are subtle or invisible on radiographs, the diagnosis is made based upon discrete tenderness on the distal radius and not elsewhere. Lister's tubercle dorsally and the radial styloid volarly provide useful landmarks to confirm what you are pressing on. A wrist sprain will be tender over the dorsal ulnar aspect of the wrist more distally, and radiographs often show a small avulsion fracture from the triquetrum.

Open wounds associated with dorsally displaced fractures are usually pinpoint volar-ulnar wounds caused by the proximal/shaft fragment. Sometimes, the wound is more substantial and more ulnar—a type of tearing of the skin with protrusion of the ulnar head (Figure 13-2). With a volarly displaced fracture, the shaft can create a small wound dorsally (Figure 13-3)—check carefully for extensor tendon injuries because you will likely use a volar exposure for débridement and internal fixation in surgery and will not directly inspect the tendons.

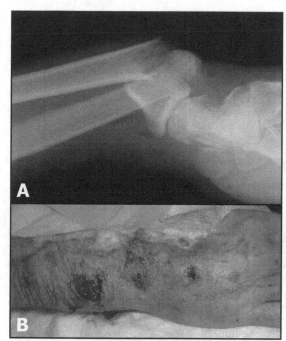

Figure 13-3. (A) Lateral radiograph of a volarly displaced fracture of the distal radius. (B) The proximal radial shaft created a dorsal wound.

HAND FRACTURES

A fractured hand is usually swollen and ecchymotic in the region of the fracture, but palpation may be needed to identify the fractured bone. One can also inspect for crepitation or instability in the obtunded patient.

Angular deformity with conversion of the fingers toward one another and rotational deformity with overlap in flexion should be identified (Figure 13-4). Active flexion is optimal, but the tenodesis effect (passive finger flexion with passive wrist extension) can help. It can also be useful to passively flex the fingers. All of this may be easier with the patient anesthetized if the fracture is quite painful. It can be difficult to evaluate rotational deformity. General guidelines are that the fingers tend to all point to the scaphoid tubercle in flexion (Figure 13-5), and the finger nails are roughly parallel, angling slightly toward the long finger (Figure 13-6). The distal interphalangeal joints tend to angle slightly toward the long finger

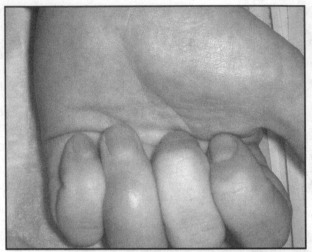

Figure 13-4. Malunion of the ring finger metacarpal creates a space between the ring and long fingers in full flexion.

Figure 13-5. To some degree, properly aligned fingers point to the distal pole of the scaphoid with the fingers flexed.

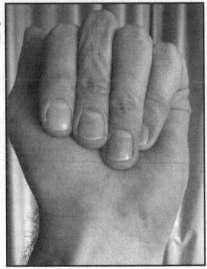

in the radioulnar plane as well (Figure 13-7). Swelling, bleeding, and incisions likely affect rotation, and it can be very difficult to assess after fixation.

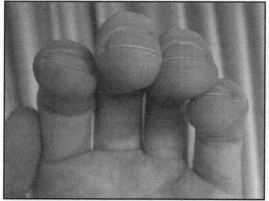

Figure 13-6. The alignment of the fingernails in extension is a less reliable guide to rotation. The index finger rotates somewhat toward the thumb, but the ring and small finger rotate somewhat toward the long finger.

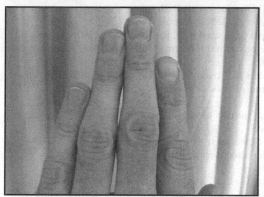

Figure 13-7. Ulnar Impaction Lesion of the lunate.

Conclusion

Physical examination provides important information in the management of fractures. Familiarity with surface anatomy, provocative tests, and other aspects of the examination can facilitate and improve management of fractures in the arm.

REFERENCES

1. Hotchkiss RN. Fractures and dislocations of the elbow. In: Rockwood CA, Green DP, Bucholz RW, Heckman JD, editors. *Rockwood and Green's Fractures in Adults, Fourth Edition.* Philadelphia: Lippincott-Raven; 1996:929-1024.
2. O'Driscoll SW, Morrey BF, Korinek S, An KN. Elbow subluxation and dislocation. A spectrum of instability. *Clin Orthop.* 1992;280:186-197.
3. Coonrad RW, Roush TF, Major NM, Basamania CJ. The drop sign, a radiographic warning sign of elbow instability. *J Shoulder Elbow Surg.* 2005;14(3):312-317.
4. Duckworth AD, Kulijdian A, McKee MD, Ring D. Residual subluxation of the elbow after dislocation or fracture-dislocation: Treatment with active elbow exercises and avoidance of varus stress. *J Shoulder Elbow Surg.* 2008;17(2):276-280.
5. O'Driscoll SW, Bell DF, Morrey BF. Posterolateral rotatory instability of the elbow. *J Bone Joint Surg.* 1991;73A:440-446.
6. Smith AM, Urbanosky LR, Castle JA, Rushing JT, Ruch DS. Radius pull test: predictor of longitudinal forearm instability. *J Bone Joint Surg Am.* 2002;84A:1970-1976.
7. O'Driscoll SW, Jupiter JB, Cohen M, Ring D, McKee MD. Difficult elbow fractures: Pearls and pitfalls. *Instructional Course Lectures.* 2003;52:113-134.
8. Ring D. Fractures of the coronoid process of the ulna. *J Hand Surg [Am].* 2006;31(10):1679-1689.
9. Ring D. Apparent capitellar fractures. *Hand Clin.* 2007;23(4):471-479, vii.
10. Shin R, Ring D. The ulnar nerve in elbow trauma. *J Bone Joint Surg Am.* 2007;89(5):1108-1116.
11. Parvizi J, Wayman J, Kelly P, Moran CG. Combining the clinical signs improves diagnosis of scaphoid fractures. A prospective study with follow-up. *J Hand Surg Br.* 1998;23(3):324-327.
12. Ring D, Lozano-Calderon S. Imaging for suspected scaphoid fracture. *J Hand Surg Am.* 2008;33(6):954-957.

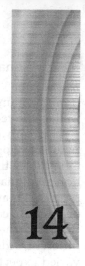

14

WOUNDS AND SOFT-TISSUE INJURIES

Jeffrey B. Friedrich, MD, FACS

INTRODUCTION

The soft-tissue envelope of the elbow, wrist, and hand is uniquely designed to allow an almost unlimited array of motor functions while providing tactile input from the surrounding environment. Additionally, the hands—much like the face—are associated with identity, and as such, there is an aesthetic component involved with the soft tissue of the upper extremity. Because of these 2 paradigms (function and form), any compromise in the upper extremity soft tissue has

Culp RW, Jacoby SM. *Musculoskeletal Examination of the Elbow, Wrist, and Hand: Making the Complex Simple* (pp. 291-309). © 2012 Taylor & Francis Group.

significant implications in terms of the wounds themselves, as well as the reconstruction of these wounds.

There are a number of insults that can compromise the soft-tissue envelope of the hand, wrist, and elbow. The most common forces that disrupt the soft tissue include trauma, infection, malignancy, and thermal injury. While each one of these problems may result in a similar-appearing defect in the hand or forearm, each individual mechanism has associated factors that make the evaluation and management of the problem very different. Additionally, each patient is unique and will have varied expectations regarding his or her needs and wants for the restoration of both form and function of the extremity.

HISTORY

The history of a compromise in the soft tissue of the upper extremity is of paramount importance for both wound evaluation and reconstruction planning. There is not a catch-all inventory of history points that is used to assess patients. Rather, the aspects of the history are dictated by the mechanism of injury to, or compromise of, the soft tissue. Pertinent historical points are listed below by general mechanism of injury.

Trauma

The actual mechanism by which the hand or arm was injured is perhaps the single most important factor that can be gleaned from the history. These are generally classified as sharp cuts (saws, knives); crushes (machinery, doors, heavy objects); avulsions (ropes, chains); gunshots, blasts (fireworks); and injuries with aspects of multiple mechanisms (such as lawnmowers that can induce both a slicing and a crushing component). The time elapsed between injury and evaluation is also important, especially when dealing with ischemic tissues. The contamination of the injury environment will help guide efforts of infection prophylaxis and control.

Infection

Vector of infection (if known) will be very helpful to guide initial management, especially when initiating empiric antibiotics. Vectors can include bites (animal or human); lacerations, punctures (needles, nails); hematogenous spread; or idiopathic vector. Location of infection nidus is important to document, as adequate infection treatment requires treatment at its "epicenter." Rapidity of progression of the infection, as well as constitutional symptoms (fevers, chills, nausea) will give clues to the severity of the infection. Patient history of immunocompromising diseases will also impact infection management.

Malignancy

Important factors to know about potential or known malignancies of the upper extremity include duration of tumor, rate of growth, pain associated with the tumor, known prior malignancy, history of sun exposure, and any constitutional symptoms since tumor development.

Thermal Injury

Like traumatic injuries, thermal injury treatment relies, in part, on the type of thermal injury. These include flame/flash burn, contact burn, electrical injury, chemical burn, or steam burn. Time elapsed since injury will also impact management.

In addition to the mechanism-related factors listed, it will be crucial to obtain other information from the patient, such as medical problems that could impact circulation or wound healing, and personal issues such as smoking or recreational drug usage.

EXAMINATION

To adequately examine the soft tissue of the upper extremity, all dressings, casts, and splints should be removed. The patient may require pain medication prior to this exam because dressing and bandage removal can be painful when open wounds are present. Long-sleeved shirts should either be removed or the sleeves rolled up. Good lighting in the examining environment should be ensured, particularly because examination of the soft tissue of the upper extremity is primarily visual.

Table 14-1

Methods of Examination

Examination	Technique	Grading	Significance
Scarring	Observation, palpation	Normal	Normal
		Hypertrophic	Abnormal
		Keloid	Abnormal
Scar contracture	Observation, palpation	Distinct band	Can be treated with local rearrangment
		Broad scar	Treated with incision, skin grafting
Open wounds	Observation, palpation, smell	Granulation	Normal
		No granulation	Poor/chronic wound healing
		Exposed structures (nerve, tendon, bone, hardware)	Requires flap coverage

The soft tissue of the hand, wrist, and elbow is observed (Table 14-1). One should make note of healed wounds, if present. The visual appearance of the scar is important, as well as its feel to the touch. Most scars, when mature, will be flat, soft, and thin. However, hypertrophic scarring (scar is raised but confined to the wound itself) and keloid scarring (scar is raised and has grown beyond the original scar) can be thick and firm to the touch. Any tight, contracted scars should be noted, including their relationship and proximity to nearby joints. If the scar is contracted, one should note whether it has caused a distinct linear scar band or a broad scar with no distinct bands (Figures 14-1 and 14-2). It is also essential that these healed wounds be examined in a dynamic state (eg, how a scar crossing the antecubital fossa reacts to flexion and extension of the elbow). Finally, scar "stability" should be assessed. Scar instability is manifested as scabbing and epidermal desquamation due to repeated cracking and opening of the scar with movement. Patients will often relate that the scar "breaks open" or "cracks" when it is unstable.

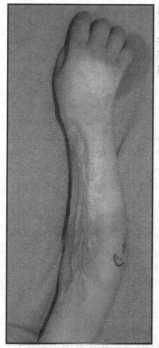

Figure 14-1. Arm and forearm following free-flap reconstruction for a severe avulsion injury. Note the tight scar band on the forearm dorsum. This scar band limits the patient's elbow extension.

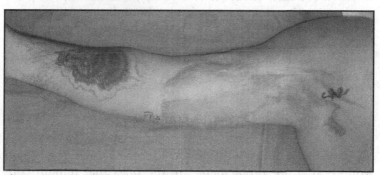

Figure 14-2. Antecubital fossa scarring following crush injury to the arm. The arm wound was initially skin grafted, which led to a broad contracture over the antecubital fossa that limited elbow extension.

When open wounds are present, the tissue that is exposed is inspected visually. Exposed structures such as nerves, vessels, tendons, bone, and hardware are noted. The presence and quality of granulation tissue in a wound that is older than 5 to 7 days can give clues to the health of the wound. Granulation tissue is a normal mix of collagen, fibrinogen, bacteria, and new blood vessels that forms in the vascularized portion of wounds. Poor or absent granulation tissue in areas that should normally generate granulation can be a sign of pathologic wound healing due to immunosuppression, radiation, infection, diminished vascularity, or residual necrotic tissue. Discharge or fluid in the wound is also taken into account. It may sound unusual, but the odor of the wound can also be helpful in assessment. A healthy healing wound should be odorless, but one with a musty or foul smell can signal infection or inadequate débridement.

The soft tissue adjacent to the open wound is also inspected. One must note any edema, ecchymosis, erythema, maceration, or pallor. The capillary refill of adjacent skin allows some assessment of the tissue vascularity. Like healed scars, the open wound's proximity to joints will also potentially help guide management.

Soft-tissue masses or tumors can occur in the upper extremity with regularity. These are most commonly benign in nature. Any mass of the hand, wrist, or forearm must be assessed for size, tenderness, mobility, relationship to joint, overlying skin changes, drainage, boundaries (distinct or indistinct), compressibility, and transillumination. When there is any concern for malignancy, the patient should be examined for the presence of pathologic (greater than 1 cm) epitrochlear or axillary lymph nodes.

PATHOANATOMY

All healed wounds will contract to some degree. The healed wounds that are problematic are the ones that remain contracted over time, despite scar modification measures such as massage, taping, and silicone application. When contracted, these scars can be symptomatic, especially with movement. Most contracted scars will manifest as distinct linear bands or cords when the affected area is brought out to length with joint extension.

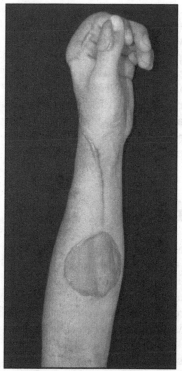

Figure 14-3. Hand and forearm following thumb and index finger reconstruction using a radial forearm fasciocutaneous flap. Note the hypertrophic scarring at the wrist.

Wounds that heal by secondary intention or those that have been skin grafted tend to form broader contractures (see Figure 14-2). When the joint is extended, there are no distinct bands. Rather, the entire area is tight and limits motion. At times, there are healed wounds that exhibit characteristics of both types of scarring (bands and broad scars).

Scars themselves can demonstrate "pathologic" healing, leading them to be symptomatic.[1] The most common type of abnormal healing is hypertrophic scarring, in which the scar is raised and tight but does not expand beyond the boundaries of the scar (Figure 14-3). Keloid scarring happens when the scar grows beyond the original boundaries of the wound and results in a bulbous or pedunculated scar. Both of these types of abnormal scarring are more common in dark-skinned individuals and are uncommon in the upper extremity.

Any type of open wound is, by default, pathologic. However, secondary pathology can be a factor with these wounds and can result in infection or poor wound healing. Poor quality or chronic wounds will have a paucity of granulation tissue and little evidence of epithelialization at the wound margins. Infected wounds may have surrounding erythema, discharge, or a foul odor. It is important to note that while a wound may not appear infected, it may contain enough bacterial colonies to classify it as infected. This can be determined with quantitative culture. Colony counts greater than 10^6 are considered infected and warrant treatment.

IMAGING

There are few imaging studies that are helpful for upper-extremity soft-tissue pathology. Computed tomography (CT) scans can be somewhat helpful in assessing a soft-tissue lesion's relationship to other structures, particularly the skeletal structures of the upper extremity. When combined with intravenous contrast, CTs can have some utility in the diagnosis of infections.

When dealing with soft tissues of the upper extremity, magnetic resonance imaging (MRI) likely yields the greatest benefit to diagnostic efforts, particularly when assessing soft-tissue masses.[2,3] While it is no substitute for tissue sampling, an MRI can be helpful in determining the general composition of a soft-tissue mass (solid or fluid filled). When combined with contrast (MR angiography), MRI can yield valuable information for vessel-based masses such as vascular malformations.

TREATMENT

Please refer to Table 14-2 for concise wound and scar treatment strategies.

Scar Contractures

As stated previously, the most important determination to make when assessing symptomatic upper extremity scars is whether the scarring is linear and distinct or if it is broad.

Table 14-2

Helpful Hints

WOUND PROBLEM	MANAGEMENT OF PROBLEM	RATIONALE
Wounds		
Wound with exudate	1. Wet to dry dressings or dressings with enzymatic debrider 2. Surgical débridement	Wounds that have exudate or other nonviable tissue require some form of débridement prior to coverage or healing by secondary intent.
Moist or draining wound	1. Negative pressure dressing 2. Surgical débridement	Negative pressure dressings work well to control wound fluid, although consider débridement as a persistently draining wound can indicate residual nonviable tissue.
Clean granulating wound	1. Negative pressure dressing 2. Petroleum-based dressings	A clean wound needs only to be kept moist. Negative pressure dressings can eliminate the need for daily dressing changes. ***Caution:*** Prolonged negative pressure dressing application causes severe tissue induration and scarring, complicating later reconstruction.
Wound with exposed "white" or "silver" structures (nerve, tendon, bone, hardware)	Wound closure or reconstruction	Exposed structures or hardware will never granulate, even with negative pressure dressings. Therefore, ensure there are no undue delays to wound closure.

(continued)

Table 14-2 (continued)

Helpful Hints

WOUND PROBLEM	MANAGEMENT OF PROBLEM	RATIONALE
Scars		
Tight scar contracture	Consider scar release and tissue rearrangement or skin grafting	Scar contractures over joints can limit range of motion in the upper extremity.
Hypertrophic scar (enlarged scar that does not exceed original scar boundaries)	1. Pressure application (massage, taping) 2. Steroid injection 3. Silicone application (tape or gel)	Many modalities have been tried, but pressure application, silicone, and steroid injections have been repeatedly shown to have benefit for hypertrophic scars.
Keloid scar (enlarged scar that exceeds boundaries of original scar)	1. As above for hypertrophic scar 2. Consider scar excision	True keloid scars are rare on the hand and are more common on the shoulders and chest.

Linear scar contractures are effectively treated with scar-tissue rearrangement. There are several techniques for scar revision. The most common technique is the Z-plasty. This method uses adjacent tissue to gain length in the scar. The middle limb of the "Z" is the scar itself, and there are 2 parallel incisions made from either end of the scar. These incisions are typically made at 60 degrees to the original scar but can be made at more obtuse angles to gain more scar lengthening. The drawback to increased scar lengthening is that more tissue from the sides must be used. This can be difficult in areas with little adjacent tissue such as the fingers. Rather than making one very large Z-plasty, a number of smaller Z-plasties can be combined to gain a similar amount of scar lengthening. These Z-plasty combinations are often sequential along the length of the scar. Additionally, 2 Z-plasties can be combined in either a double-opposing fashion or a 4-flap Z-plasty in order to gain more scar lengthening (Figure 14-4). These 2 techniques are particularly useful for the revision of first webspace post-traumatic contractures.

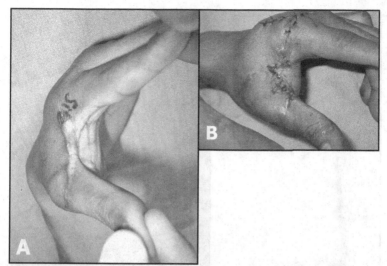

Figure 14-4. (A) First webspace contracture, which limited thumb abduction. (B) This was treated with a double-opposing Z-plasty procedure.

When scarring is broad and there are no distinct bands or cords, revision is typically accomplished with scar incision followed by application of a full-thickness or split-thickness skin graft into the defect that is created (Figure 14-5). In the hand, these grafts are usually full-thickness, while they are typically split-thickness in the forearm and antecubital fossa.

Open Wounds

Perhaps the most common soft-tissue problem that a hand or upper-extremity surgeon may be called upon to treat is an open wound. As stated before, these wounds can be caused by a variety of inciting factors, including trauma, thermal injury, infection, or malignancy. The first priority of wound reconstruction is thorough removal of the inciting disease process. In traumatic wounds, this requires débridement of any foreign or necrotic material. In thermal injury, it is imperative to remove all devitalized skin prior to skin grafting. Infections must be adequately drained or debrided prior to coverage. Finally, complete excision of a malignancy must be ensured prior to soft-tissue reconstruction.

Primary closure and healing by secondary intention are the easiest methods to close soft tissue in the upper extremity.

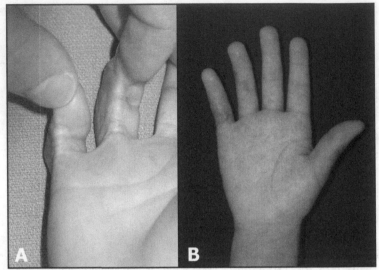

Figure 14-5. (A) Flexion contractures of the ring and small finger following thermal injury. (B) The ringer finger was treated with Z-plasties, while the small finger (more severe of the two) was treated with scar incision and full-thickness skin grafting.

Primary closure can be employed following trauma when there is minimal or no skin loss. A small defect from excision of skin malignancy (such as squamous cell carcinoma) may also be amenable to primary closure if there is enough skin laxity. Healing by secondary intent can be safely employed in small wounds when there are no exposed vital structures such as tendons, nerves, or vessels. This method is often used following infection or contaminated traumatic wounds.

Negative pressure dressings have become an important adjunct in the management of wounds of the hand.[4,5,6] It must be emphasized that basic wound management principles cannot be abandoned and should precede usage of this type of dressing. Thorough débridement of all contaminated and devitalized tissue is mandatory prior to negative pressure-dressing placement. While these dressings are not substitutes for proper wound management, they may allow surgeons to use a less complex wound closure method than would have been the case without the negative pressure dressing (eg, ability to cover a wound with a skin graft rather than a vascularized flap).

Skin grafts are an important component of upper-extremity wound treatment. These can be used when no "vital" structures, such as nerves, vessels, or tendons, are exposed. Additionally, the base of the wound itself must be well-vascularized because the skin graft will initially survive on nutrient and oxygen diffusion from the wound itself. Full-thickness grafts are used on the hand because they have a lower tendency for secondary contracture and exhibit better sensory reinnervation than split grafts. The disadvantage of full-thickness grafts is that their donor sites must be closed primarily, thereby limiting the amount of skin that can be harvested. For larger hand wounds, or for more proximal wounds, split-thickness grafts are appropriate. The donor site for a split-thickness graft will heal by secondary intention. The disadvantage of any skin graft is the appearance because the color match is often not exact, and if the graft is meshed prior to placement, it can be fairly unattractive.

Because of the paucity of soft tissue in the upper extremity, particularly in the hand, open wounds will often be accompanied by exposed structures that will neither heal by secondary intent nor accept a skin graft. These structures include bone, tendon, nerves, and hardware. In these cases, a flap is warranted.[7,8] A flap is a tissue transfer that contains it own blood supply and consists of one or more types of tissue (cutaneous, fasciocutaneous, musculocutaneous, fascia, etc). There are a seemingly endless number of flaps that can be used in the upper extremity. The most common, useful flaps are as follows.

Fingers

Open wounds to the fingers, especially the tips, are very common. The donors for finger wounds can be classified as homodigital, heterodigital, and hand based.

Homodigital: There are few homodigital flaps that are useful because of the limited soft tissue of the finger.[9] The homodigital island flap can be distally based and can reach the fingertips. A wound near the base of the digit can be closed with an axial flag flap. The adipofascial flap is a flap from the proximal end of the digit that is used to close fingertip wounds. It is an axial flap based on the dorsal digital circulation.

Heterodigital: The cross-finger flap is perhaps the most useful heterodigital flap. This flap uses tissue from the dorsum of an adjacent digit to cover a palmar wound. A cross-finger flap from the index finger can cover the thumb. The reverse-cross finger flap employs the adipofascial layer from the dorsum of a digit to cover a wound on the dorsum of the adjacent digit. All cross-finger flaps require skin grafting of the donor or recipient site and require flap division 2 to 3 weeks later.

Hand based: The index and middle fingertips can be reconstructed with a thenar flap. This is a random-pattern flap from the thenar eminence that is elevated and sutured to the digit tip. The disadvantages of this flap are the necessity of flap division 2 to 3 weeks later and the proximal interphalangeal (PIP) joint contracture that can result from flexion of this joint prior to flap division. The dorsal metacarpal artery system has become an invaluable resource for hand and digit reconstruction.[10] The proximally based versions of these flaps are perfused by the dorsal metacarpal arteries themselves. All are reliable except the fourth dorsal metacarpal artery. The distally based version of the flap is perfused by a palmar-dorsal vascular connection at the level of the metacarpal neck. The flap can be fasciocutaneous or fascia only. They are able to reach the thumb and fingertips (Figure 14-6). The versatility of these flaps exceed that of other hand-based flaps.

Hand

It is rare to encounter a hand defect that warrants flap closure and can be closed by local tissue. The fillet of finger flap has some utility in covering the dorsal hand in cases where the soft tissue of the digit is viable but the digit itself is not salvageable (Figure 14-7).[11] Other than those rare cases, one must look elsewhere for donor tissue. Forearm-based flaps can be extremely useful for hand wound coverage and can reach the fingers. The most common of these is the radial forearm flap (see Figure 14-3). This flap is based on reversed flow in the radial artery by way of the palmar arch and ulnar artery. It is imperative to perform an Allen test prior to this transfer to confirm that the ulnar artery will adequately perfuse all digits of the hand once the radial artery is divided proximally. Different permutations of the flap can be used, including fasciocutaneous, fascia alone, suprafascial, and even as a perforator flap, which allows preservation of the radial artery proper.[12,13] While the advantages of the radial forearm flap are considerable, it does have disadvantages. There can be cold intolerance, presumably from sacrifice of the radial artery, and

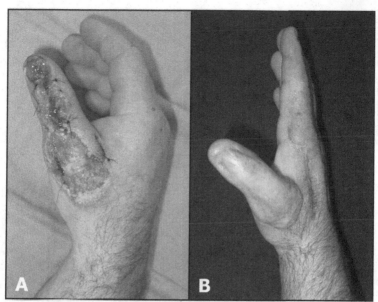

Figure 14-6. (A) Dorsal thumb avulsion injury. (B) This was treated with a proximally based dorsal metacarpal artery flap from the index ray. The donor site was covered with a full-thickness skin graft.

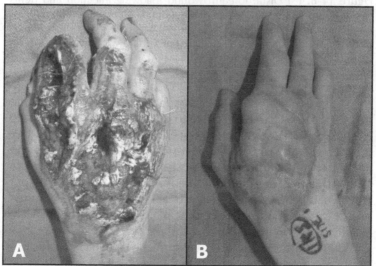

Figure 14-7. (A) Mangling injury of the dorsal hand. The index finger musculoskeletal units were damaged beyond salvage, but the volar skin of the finger was uninjured. (B) This index finger soft tissue was transferred as a fillet flap to cover the dorsal hand.

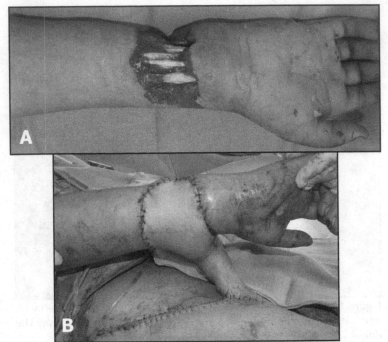

Figure 14-8. (A) Distal forearm wound following infection and dehiscence of a primarily closed traumatic wound. A radial forearm flap was contraindicated because the radial artery was the only perfusing vessel of the hand. (B) Therefore, a pedicled groin flap was used to cover the wound.

the skin-grafted donor site can be fairly ugly if a fasciocutaneous flap is used. An alternative to the radial forearm flap is the posterior interosseous artery flap. Like the radial forearm flap, it is perfused by retrograde perfusion, which is via anastomoses between the anterior and posterior interosseous arteries.[14] While this flap sacrifices no major artery to the hand, its perfusion can be tenuous if the pedicle is near the zone of injury, and it can have a donor site that is not particularly attractive when covered with a skin graft.

When there are factors that prevent transfer of a local or regional flap, the pedicled groin flap is an excellent option.[15,16] An enormous piece of well-vascularized tissue can be transferred to the hand or wrist (Figure 14-8). The vascular supply to the flap is robust and is rarely compromised. The flap donor site can be closed primarily, simply by flexing the hip and/or putting the operating table in flexion. The disadvantages of the flap are its bulk and the attachment of the hand to the groin for 2 to 3 weeks while vascular ingrowth from the hand to the flap occurs. Because of this vascular ingrowth period, a second surgery to divide the pedicle is obligatory. It is not unusual for the groin flap to require debulking, even in slender patients. This debulking can be performed by direct fat excision or liposuction.

There are the occasional upper extremity wounds that are too large or too complicated to be adequately treated with local, regional, or distant pedicled flaps. In those cases, free-tissue transfer is required.[17] The transfer of these flaps does require microsurgical expertise, but in the current era, it is reasonable to expect free flap survival rates in excess of 95% at experienced centers. Free muscle flaps are relied upon heavily for coverage in other parts of the body such as the trunk and lower extremity. However, with few exceptions— such as the serratus anterior free flap—muscle flaps are too bulky for the hand, even following post-transfer muscle atrophy. In these cases, it is reasonable to transfer fasciocutaneous flaps or fascia flaps that are covered with skin grafts. Acceptable free fasciocutaneous flap donors include the contralateral radial forearm flap, dorsalis pedis flap, and the lateral arm flap. The lateral arm flap is particularly useful because it has a reliable pedicle of reasonable length, does not require sacrifice of a major artery, and can be harvested from the ipsilateral arm.[18] The donor site can be somewhat unattractive if closed with a skin graft. There are several flaps that work well as fascia-alone transfers that are covered by skin grafts. This type of flap construct works well on the dorsal hand because there is no excess bulk. These flaps include the fasciocutaneous donors listed above, as well as the temporoparietal fascia flap and the anterolateral thigh fascia flap.[19] In more proximal areas such as the forearm and elbow, fasciocutaneous flaps and muscle flaps can be used because the issue of flap bulk is not as great a concern as it is in the hand. Suitable muscle flaps for the forearm and elbow include the rectus abdominis flap, the gracilis flap, and, in cases of enormous tissue loss, the latissimus dorsi flap (Figure 14-9).

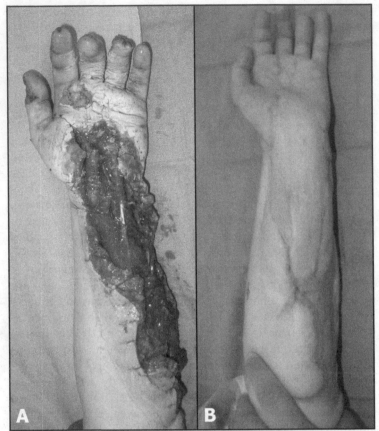

Figure 14-9. (A) Severe mangling injury of the volar forearm and wrist. There are no local options to cover this wound, and a groin flap is inadequate. (B) This wound was reconstructed with a free gracilis muscle flap that was simultaneously covered with split-thickness skin grafts.

CONCLUSION

The examination of the soft tissue of the upper extremity requires knowledge about the disease process affecting each particular patient. The etiology of the soft-tissue problem guides initial management and later reconstruction. There are a number of sound techniques that can be used to treat both open and closed soft-tissue abnormalities of the upper extremity.

REFERENCES

1. Niessen FB, Spauwen PH, Schalkwijk J, Kon M. On the nature of hypertrophic scars and keloids: a review. *Plast Reconstr Surg.* 1999;104(5):1435-1458.
2. Stacy GS, Nair L. Magnetic resonance imaging features of extremity sarcomas of uncertain differentiation. *Clin Radiol.* 2007;62(10):950-958.
3. Teh J, Whiteley G. MRI of soft tissue masses of the hand and wrist. *Br J Radiol.* 2007;80(949):47-63.
4. Geiger S, McCormick F, Chou R, Wandel AG. War wounds: lessons learned from Operation Iraqi Freedom. *Plast Reconstr Surg.* 2008;122(1):146-153.
5. Kairinos N, Solomons M, Hudson DA. Negative-pressure wound therapy I: the paradox of negative-pressure wound therapy. *Plast Reconstr Surg.* 2009;123(2):589-598; discussion 599-600.
6. Kairinos N, Voogd AM, Botha PH, et al. Negative-pressure wound therapy II: negative-pressure wound therapy and increased perfusion. Just an illusion? *Plast Reconstr Surg.* 2009;123(2):601-612.
7. Levin LS. Principles of definitive soft tissue coverage with flaps. *J Orthop Trauma.* 2008;22(10 Suppl):S161-S166.
8. Trumble TT, Vedder NB. Tissue transfer: Pedicle and free tissue flaps. In: Trumble TT, ed. Principles of hand surgery and therapy. Philadelphia: WB Saunders; 2000:499-528.
9. Bickel KD, Dosanjh A. Fingertip reconstruction. *J Hand Surg [Am].* 2008;33(8):1417-1419.
10. Gregory H, Heitmann C, Germann G. The evolution and refinements of the distally based dorsal metacarpal artery (DMCA) flaps. *J Plast Reconstr Aesthet Surg.* 2007;60(7):731-739.
11. Kuntscher MV, Erdmann D, Homann HH, Steinau HU, Levin SL, Germann G. The concept of fillet flaps: classification, indications, and analysis of their clinical value. *Plast Reconstr Surg.* 2001;108(4):885-896.
12. Page R, Chang J. Reconstruction of hand soft-tissue defects: alternatives to the radial forearm fasciocutaneous flap. *J Hand Surg [Am].* 2006;31(5):847-856.
13. Schaverien M, Saint-Cyr M. Suprafascial compared with subfascial harvest of the radial forearm flap: an anatomic study. *J Hand Surg [Am].* 2008;33(1):97-101.
14. Cheema TA, Lakshman S, Cheema MA, Durrani SF. Reverse-flow posterior interosseous flap: a review of 68 cases. *Hand (NY).* 2007;2(3):112-116.
15. Chow JA, Bilos ZJ, Hui P, Hall RF, Seyfer AE, Smith AC. The groin flap in reparative surgery of the hand. *Plast Reconstr Surg.* 1986;77(3):421-426.
16. Li YY, Wang JL, Lu Y, Huang J. Resurfacing deep wound of upper extremities with pedicled groin flaps. *Burns.* 2000;26(3):283-288.
17. Yildirim S, Taylan G, Eker G, Akoz T. Free flap choice for soft tissue reconstruction of the severely damaged upper extremity. *J Reconstr Microsurg.* 2006;22(8):599-609.
18. Scheker LR, Kleinert HE, Hanel DP. Lateral arm composite tissue transfer to ipsilateral hand defects. *J Hand Surg [Am].* 1987;12(5 Pt 1):665-672.
19. Wang HT, Erdmann D, Fletcher JW, Levin LS. Anterolateral thigh flap technique in hand and upper extremity reconstruction. *Tech Hand Up Extrem Surg.* 2004;8(4):257-261.

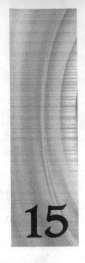

15

VASCULAR
EVALUATION OF THE
UPPER EXTREMITY

Diane Payne, MD and Marc J. Richard, MD

INTRODUCTION

Vascular disorders of the upper extremity are relatively uncommon compared to other locations in the body. These disorders significantly alter overall patient health and function. The successful evaluation and management of upper extremity vascular disorders can reduce the morbidity associated with these conditions.

Culp RW, Jacoby SM. *Musculoskeletal Examination of the Elbow, Wrist, and Hand: Making the Complex Simple* (pp. 310-327). © 2012 Taylor & Francis Group.

ANATOMY

The vessels that eventually supply the hand come from the subclavian artery and course from the thoracic cavity into the upper extremity as the axillary artery. The axillary artery then becomes the brachial artery, which gives rise to the radial and ulnar arteries, a parallel and interconnected arterial system supplying nutrition and metabolic requirements to the hand.

The ulnar artery enters the hand through Guyon's canal between the pisiform and the hook of the hamate. The ulnar artery typically lies radial to the ulnar nerve. The ulnar artery continues as the superficial palmar arch. After passing deep to the first dorsal compartment at the wrist, the radial artery enters the palm between the 2 heads of the first dorsal interosseous muscle, followed by the 2 heads of the adductor pollicis muscle to become the deep palmar arch. The superficial arch lies more distal in the palm than the deep arch. The superficial arch gives rise to 3 palmar common digital arteries, which divide again to form the proper digital arteries that run along the radial and ulnar sides of the digits. The deep palmar arch gives off 3 palmar metacarpal arteries and the princeps pollicis artery, which supplies the palmar surface of the thumb. A persistent median artery is contributory to the vascular supply of the hand in approximately 5% of patients. The arch is considered complete if there is a second contributory vessel connecting to it. The deep arch is complete in 97% of individuals, whereas only 78.5% of hands demonstrate a complete superficial arch.[1,2]

The microvascular beds of the hand are composed of those vessels that are less than 100 μm in diameter. These nutritional and thermoregulatory capillary beds are most concentrated in the superficial aspects of the digital pulps. Only 5% to 20% of the total blood flow through these microvascular beds are responsible for nutritional flow supporting cellular metabolism. The vast majority of blood flow through the microvascular beds contributes to the thermoregulatory effect of this system.[3] A wide variety of disease states affect the complex regulation of this system, resulting in symptoms ranging from cold intolerance to ischemic ulcers.

Blood flow within the hand and digits is controlled by sympathetic tone, metabolic demands, environmental events, local factors, and humeral mediators.[4] Locally or centrally released mediators can induce vasoconstriction or vasodilation of the vascular system. Metabolic autoregulation occurs at a local level, which allows the microvascular bed to match local perfusion to local metabolic needs. Environmental temperature as well as blood pressure and blood flow has an effect on increasing or decreasing perfusion through microvascular beds. For example, increased blood pressure increases wall tension, causing reflexive vasoconstriction in arteriole walls. Postural changes cause the microcirculation to limit cutaneous perfusion, thereby causing vasoconstriction to minimize limb-dependent edema.[4]

The peripheral nervous system has a large effect on microvascular control, and normal function of the microvascular system requires these nerves to be intact and functioning. Sympathetic fibers travel along the adventitia of blood vessels and innervate the arteriole and venous walls. Over-activity of these nerves can cause significant vasoconstriction, subsequently limiting flow distally.

HISTORY

Underlying medical conditions can influence the presence of vascular disease and can affect vascular perfusion to the hand. Diabetes mellitus, peripheral vascular disease, cardiac arrhythmias, connective tissue disorders, and familial or sporadic blood dyscrasias can all have profound effects on upper extremity hemodynamics. Vascular access for dialysis can alter the blood flow through the upper extremity, resulting in vascular steal phenomena. Trauma can result in direct vascular injury, while repetitive trauma and vibratory exposure can predispose to vascular occlusion and vasospastic disorders, respectively. Tobacco, caffeine, and alcohol exposure are external stimuli that can alter vascular flow.[3]

Obtaining an accurate history from the patient is vital, as the patient can direct your focused examination from the details he or she uses to describe the symptoms. Furthermore, many vascular disorders result in intermittent signs and symptoms, which may not be present when the patient is being examined in the physician's office. This places a greater importance on obtaining an accurate and complete patient history. It is important to determine if the patient sustained a trauma to his or her extremity, either penetrating or blunt. Repetitive insults to the hypothenar aspect of the hand can result in thrombosis of the ulnar artery in Guyon's canal, known as hypothenar hammer syndrome. Baseball catchers and manual laborers who use their hand as a hammer are specifically prone to this condition. The history should also assess swelling; cold intolerance; color changes; ulcers; and exposure to drugs, toxins, or tobacco. Complaints of numbness, weakness, or pain are also documented.

EVALUATION

Evaluation of the blood supply to the upper extremity requires visual, auscultatory, and palpatory assessment. An assessment of vascular sufficiency begins with visual inspection. The skin is evaluated for overall integrity, color, and the presence or absence of lesions, blisters, ulcers, or gangrene. Arterial insufficiency will produce white or grayish discoloration of affected areas and a cool digit, whereas venous abnormalities result in a purple, congested digit. Visual inspection should include the nails to evaluate for subungual splinter hemorrhages that indicate proximal arterial lesions with embolism. The vascular examination should include evaluation of capillary refill and turgor (soft-tissue pressure) at the distal fingertips. When the fingertip is compressed, it should turn pale, then regain a pink color as blood refills the digit within 2 seconds. A longer delay is an indication of vascular insufficiency (Table 15-1).[5]

Palpation or auscultation should be used to determine the quality of the brachial, radial, and ulnar pulses, specifically evaluating for any masses or bruits. The Allen test is an objective assessment of perfusion patterns of the hand.[6] The test is performed by exsanguinating blood from the hand while compressing both the ulnar and radial arteries (see Table 15-1). The patient assists by closing the hand tightly, while the examiner provides direct pressure over both arteries. The patient then

Table 15-1

Methods for Vascular Examination of the Upper Extremity

Examination	Technique	Illustration	Significance
Allen test	Blood is exsanguinated from the hand by the examiner and both the radial and ulnar arteries are occluded with compression from the examiner's thumbs. The patient's fingers are extended to a resting position. The examiner releases the ulnar artery, and the perfusion of the hand is evaluated. Information is obtained about the presence and pattern of perfusion. In the normal hand, perfusion should return in <6 seconds. The same procedure is repeated for the radial artery.	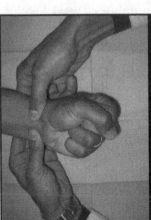	Perfusion of the entire hand with release of the ulnar or radial artery demonstrates a complete palmar arch. Incomplete perfusion is indicative of an incomplete arch, and in this case, both ulnar and radial artery flow is required to perfuse the hand and digits. Perfusion should be present in <6 seconds in the normal hand.

(continued)

Table 15-1 (continued)

Methods for Vascular Examination of the Upper Extremity

EXAMINATION	TECHNIQUE	ILLUSTRATION	SIGNIFICANCE
Allen test		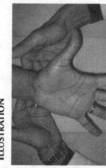	Release of the ulnar artery demonstrates reperfusion of the hand.
		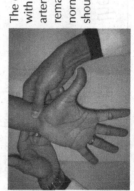	The examination is repeated with release of the ulnar artery while the radial artery remains occluded. In the normal hand, perfusion should return in <6 seconds.

(continued)

Table 15-1 (continued)

Methods for Vascular Examination of the Upper Extremity

EXAMINATION	TECHNIQUE	ILLUSTRATION	SIGNIFICANCE
Doppler examination	A handheld Doppler probe is used to assess vascular perfusion. The probe is placed directly over the vessel and provides an audible evaluation of vascular perfusion. A normal artery produces a triphasic pulsatile flow. A completely occluded vessel produces no audible response, while partial occlusion and stenosis produce monophasic flow responses.		The Doppler probe is an important tool for mapping the arterial anatomy and assessing the presence and characteristic of flow through the vessel. It can also be used in the unresponsive patient as an augment to the Allen test.
Segmental arterial pressures	Segmental artery pressures are typically obtained in the vascular laboratory by using occlusive cuffs and Doppler units to obtain systolic blood pressure measurements. Pressure ratios are compared between levels. A digital-brachial index (DBI) of >0.7 suggests adequate blood flow. A DBI of ≤0.7 suggests inadequate flow and requires intervention.		DBI > 0.7 suggests adequate vascular flow. DBI ≤ 0.7 suggests inadequate blood flow. Caution is required in interpreting segmental arterial pressures in patients with calcified vessels as this can artificially elevate the recorded pressures.

(continued)

Table 15-1 (continued)

Methods for Vascular Examination of the Upper Extremity

EXAMINATION	TECHNIQUE	ILLUSTRATION	SIGNIFICANCE
Capillary refill	(A) Depress the skin of the digital pulp with the examiner's finger (B) or the tip of a pen. Release the pressure, and evaluate the time to refill and the turgor of the skin. Refill should occur in <2 seconds, and turgor should be full. "Moving" the tip of the pen across the digital pulp can be helpful in the evaluation of appropriate refill.	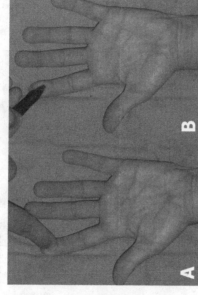	Normal skin turgor and refill in < 2 seconds is normal. Abnormal turgor or delayed/absent capillary refill is indicative of inadequate arterial perfusion.

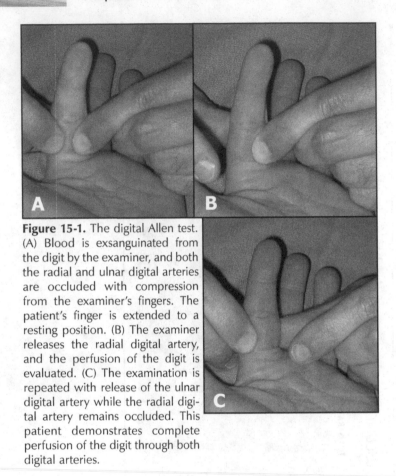

Figure 15-1. The digital Allen test. (A) Blood is exsanguinated from the digit by the examiner, and both the radial and ulnar digital arteries are occluded with compression from the examiner's fingers. The patient's finger is extended to a resting position. (B) The examiner releases the radial digital artery, and the perfusion of the digit is evaluated. (C) The examination is repeated with release of the ulnar digital artery while the radial digital artery remains occluded. This patient demonstrates complete perfusion of the digit through both digital arteries.

opens the hand with care taken not to hyperextend the wrist or digits. When the ulnar artery is released, the hand should turn pink as the blood refills into the palm within 2 to 6 seconds. If the entire palm remains pale, the ulnar artery is not patent. The order of testing can be reversed to test the radial artery. If flow is restored to only part of the hand, conclusions can be made about the completeness of the vascular arches and the perfusion pattern. The same technique can be applied to digits at the level of the proper digital arteries (Figure 15-1).

A Doppler ultrasound can be incorporated into the vascular examination if an occlusion or embolism is suspected, limiting ulnar or radial arterial flow. The device, using sound wave technology, can identify the location of the vessel obstruction distally by using sequential occlusion of the radial and ulnar arteries at the level of the wrist. Similarly, in the unexaminable patient, the Doppler can be used to document arterial perfusion patterns to the hand.[5,7]

There are a number of other noninvasive methods for evaluation of vascular flow. Pulse volume recordings (PVR) use digital plethysmography to quantify flow through an artery. Analogue tracings are produced, which quantify arterial compliance and vascular perfusion. The tracings of normal arteries produce triphasic wave patterns, whereas diseased arteries produce characteristic deviations from these patterns. PVRs are useful in differentiating vaso-occlusive from vasospastic disease as well as evaluating the effects of intervention. Furthermore, they are useful in predicting the utility of periarterial sympathectomy.[8,9]

Segmental arterial pressures are obtained by using occlusive pressure cuffs and Doppler to obtain systolic pressure measurements at various levels of the upper extremity. Large pressure differences between levels is indicative of vaso-occlusive disease. Most commonly, the digital brachial index (DBI) is obtained as a ratio of the systolic pressure of the digital artery to the systolic pressure of the brachial artery. A ratio that is 0.7 or less indicates poor perfusion, whereas greater than 0.7 indicates adequate flow. It is important to remember that calcified vessels, which can occur in diabetes mellitus, can produce falsely high pressure measurements. Vasospastic disorders do not typically result in abnormal DBIs.

Cold stress testing is used to evaluate the digital response to cold stress. This test is performed in 3 phases and provides valuable information about the autonomic and vasomotor response to and recovery from cold stress. The pulp temperature is continuously recorded at room temperature, during 20 minutes of cold immersion at 8°C, and during rewarming at room temperature for 20 minutes. Patients with abnormal responses to the cold stress test can have the test repeated after a sympathetic block with local anesthesia to help predict the potential response to surgical sympathectomy.

Finally, laboratory studies should be obtained to assess for an underlying autoimmune disease or hypercoagulable state as the potential cause of the vascular disorder. The recommended panel includes a complete blood count with differentiation, erythrocyte sedimentation rate (ESR), and C-reactive protein as markers of inflammation. Potential markers of connective tissue disorders are obtained, including rheumatoid factor, antinuclear antibody, antineutrophil cytoplasmic antibodies, antiphospholipid antibodies, serum protein electrophoresis, cryoglobulins, and complement C3 and C4 levels. The coagulopathy labs include prothrombin time, partial thrombin time, factor V leiden, protein C, protein S, and homocysteine levels.

PATHOANATOMY

Vascular disease within the upper extremity is a far less prominent entity than in the lower extremity, heart, or brain. Despite that, approximately 10% of the general population and 20% to 30% of premenopausal women will have a problem with vascular flow in the upper extremity.[4] Abnormal perfusion in the upper extremity leads to vascular insufficiency, or failure of blood flow to meet the demands of the tissue. This results in cellular ischemia, leading to cell injury and eventual cell death. This abnormal perfusion can be symptomatic, resulting in pain, cold intolerance, numbness, and digital skin changes, including eventual ulceration and gangrene.

Abnormal perfusion results from either a pre-existing congenital cause or from an acquired event. An acquired event results from trauma causing structural vessel damage, injury to the structures that innervate the vessel, or development of vasomotor dysfunction after the traumatic event. The injury to the vessel or its innervating structures can follow 1 of 2 pathways. If adequate collateral circulatory flow exists, the injury will cause minimal to no symptoms. If, however, adequate collateral flow is not present, tissue ischemia will result in both decreased perfusion and increased sympathetic tone, leading to vessel spasm. The final common pathway results in decreased tissue perfusion, leading to decreased nutritional flow and eventual cell death.

Ischemia of the Fingers

Pallor and paresthesia brought on by cold temperature are the hallmarks of Raynaud's disease. If the cause of the condition is idiopathic, it is referred to as Raynaud's disease; however, if the condition is caused by a known systemic illness, the condition is referred to as Raynaud's phenomena. It may be necessary to excise a portion of the sympathetic nerves in order to treat this condition, allowing dilation of the digital vessels.

Joint dislocation, fracture or crush, or penetrating trauma can result in vascular occlusion in the upper extremity and hand. This occlusion of flow can lead to development of a compartment syndrome, progressive thrombosis, or distal embolism within the hand or forearm. Because of the additional injury that accompanies the arterial injury, symptoms may be delayed or missed until the combination of intimal injury, swelling of the tissues, and hypotension to the tissues causes thrombosis. Any expansive or pulsatile hematoma should raise awareness of a vascular injury, as should absent or diminished peripheral pulses. When inadequate circulation exists, digital ischemia will ensue, resulting in an increase in sympathetic tone, causing additional vasoconstriction and further decrease in tissue perfusion. The end result of this cascade is an escalation of symptoms. When adequate flow is lacking, vascular reconstruction should be performed.

When blunt trauma is the initial insult, vascular aneurysms can result. These can be false or true aneurysms. False aneurysms are those that occur with penetration of the vessel wall resulting in hemorrhage. This hemorrhage will consolidate, fibrose, and eventually recannulate, so the lumen of the false aneurysm remains in continuity with the true vessel, but it lacks an endothelial lining. True aneurysms occur after an injury to the vessel that allows gradual vessel dilation. Both of these aneurysms occur slowly, with the end result being thrombosis. Clinical diagnosis is often made by the presence of distal ischemia, secondary to embolization, or a palpable mass. Treatment would include ligation and resection if the occurrence is in a noncritical vessel or excision of the damaged wall or the vessel with patch grafting or end-to-end repair or interpositional grafting.[3,10,11]

Occlusive disease occurs most commonly in the ulnar artery at the superficial volar arch. Hypothenar hammer syndrome, or occlusion of the ulnar arch secondary to thrombosis, is common in the older male and usually occurs secondary to repetitive trauma. The internal wall of the vessel is damaged, resulting in aneurysmal dilation, formation of thrombi, potential showering of distal emboli, or complete arterial occlusion. Treatment of this entity involves discontinuation of tobacco and altering repetitive behavior. Beyond this, pharmacological intervention including calcium channel blockers, resection and ligation or reconstruction of the damaged artery, and possible sympathectomy may be necessary.[8]

A hemangioma is a firm mass that can be bright red, blue, or normal flesh color. The growth of these tumors can slow over time and are often associated with dilated adjacent veins. Most of these will resolve by 7 years of age. It is important to distinguish simple hemangiomas from arterial vascular malformations. They can also occur with thrombocytopenia (Kasabach-Merritt syndrome), which could be life threatening. In this case, the hemangiomas need to be treated with steroids or local excision.[3]

A glomus is an arteriovenous (AV) anastomosis that helps to control skin circulation locally and is located in the dermal layer of the distal tip of the finger. Glomus cells are large round cells that surround these AV channels. A glomus tumor is a mass of these cells that form beneath the nailplate and cause significant pain, pinpoint tenderness, and cold sensitivity. These can sometimes be seen as small blue spots beneath the nail and can often be seen with transillumination of the fingertip. These tumors can be excised, taking care to protect the nail matrix.

Raynaud's phenomena is a vasospastic state with an undefined etiology (Table 15-2). It results in vasospasm of the distal digital arteries secondary to sympathetic nerve overactivity. The digit turns white secondary to ischemia, followed by blue as the tissue becomes cyanotic. The digit will then turn red as the reactive hyperemia from rebound vasodilatation occurs. Both physical exam and digital Allen testing helps to make the diagnosis. This entity is often associated with collagen vascular disease, so diagnostic studies should be performed when this is suspected. Treatment includes cessation of smoking,

Table 15-2

Helpful Hints

FEATURE	RAYNAUD'S PHENOMENON	RAYNAUD'S DISEASE
History		
Triphasic color change	Yes	Yes
Age >40 years	Yes	No
Rapid progression	Yes	No
Associated disease process	Yes	No
Female predominance	Occasional	Frequent
Physical Examination		
Abnormal Allen test	Frequent	No
Unilateral findings	Frequent	Infrequent
Trophic changes	Frequent	Infrequent
Laboratory tests		
Blood chemistry abnormalities	Frequently abnormal	Normal
Angiography abnormalities	Frequently abnormal	Normal

avoidance of cold environments that prompt vasoconstriction, and medication to block sympathetic hyperactivity. Surgical treatment can include sympathectomies to reduce vasoconstriction.

Thromboangiitis obliterans (Buerger's disease) is an occlusive disorder of small and medium vessels in the digits that begins distally and moves proximally. This disease primarily affects male smokers and they present with rest pain, claudication, and eventual ulceration. Smoking cessation is the primary treatment for this disease, and failure to do so can result in amputation of the digits as necrosis results.

IMAGING

Magnetic resonance angiography (MRA) provides visualization of the vascular anatomy of the upper extremity. Imaging can be obtained in both low- and high-flow states, giving information about velocity of flow and volume of flow. This imaging technique, when used with the administration of gadolinium through a peripheral intravenous catheter, characterizes vascular anomalies in relation to the structures that surround it. When MRA is performed using rapid sequence imaging techniques, information regarding flow patterns can be obtained. Overall, the role for MRA in evaluation of upper-extremity vascular pathology is continuing to be defined.

Computed tomography angiography (CTA) similarly provides anatomic evaluation of the vascular system of the upper extremity in relation to the surrounding osseous and soft-tissue structures. Contrast can be administered through a peripheral IV to enhance the vascular structures, and selective digital subtraction can be used to provide greater detail of the desired anatomy. The structural and functional information provided by CTA makes it a useful tool in the evaluation of the upper-extremity vascular system.

Standard contrast arteriography is the gold standard for the diagnosis of vascular pathology in the upper extremity (Figure 15-2). This technique uses statically acquired images after the administration of contrast material, typically through catheterization of the arterial system at the groin. Rapid imaging sequences provide dynamic information about blood flow and collateral vessels. Arteriography can also be used therapeutically for embolization of malformations or for catheter-directed thrombolysis of acute occlusions. Because of the need

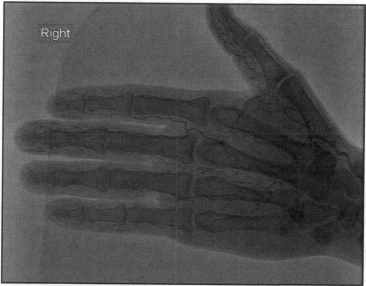

Figure 15-2. An arteriogram of a patient with hypothenar hammer syndrome. Complete occlusion of the ulnar artery in Guyon's canal is demonstrated. There is also embolization to the ring finger with resultant ischemia.

for arterial cannulation, the risks of arteriography are greater than those associated with MRA or CTA.

TREATMENT

Treatment is directed at the specific vascular disorder identified. Management strategies include pharmacologic agents, activity or environmental modifications, and surgical intervention. The treatments for some common vascular disorders are outlined below.

Acute arterial injury is evaluated for collateral circulation resulting in adequate tissue perfusion. If there is evidence of distal ischemia as demonstrated by decreased capillary refill, loss of turgor, DBI ≤ 0.7, or Allen test > 6 seconds, consideration should be given to arterial reconstruction. If there is laceration to a noncritical vessel or if there is adequate collateral circulation, ligation of the lacerated vessel is recommended. This is largely dependent upon the clinical judgment of the operating surgeon. If the arterial laceration is in the brachial artery or proximal, the vessel is routinely repaired or reconstructed.[12]

The most common form of post-traumatic occlusive disease is ulnar artery thrombosis at the proximal aspect of the superficial palmar arch known as hypothenar hammer syndrome. It is most common in laborers who use their hand as a hammer and has been reported in baseball catchers due to the repetitive impact of the baseball onto the hypothenar aspect of the hand. The pathophysiology of this condition involves disruption of the internal elastic lamina with subsequent aneurysm formation and the development of mural thrombi. These thrombi may result in occlusion of the ulnar artery or may embolize distally, most commonly into the ring finger.

The management of symptomatic ulnar artery thrombosis is again based on physical examination findings. Evaluation of the collateral circulation and the sympathetic tone are useful in the development of a successful treatment strategy. Symptoms are managed by increasing the collateral flow, regulating the sympathetic tone, or restoring the anatomic flow. Collateral flow can be increased by minimizing environmental factors that produce vasoconstriction. Avoidance of cold exposure, cessation of tobacco products, and limiting caffeine use are all recommended. The use of biofeedback and oral calcium-channel blockers (nifedipine) can also be useful. Sympathetic tone can be surgically regulated by periarterial sympathectomy or by resection and ligation of the thrombosed segment (Leriche sympathectomy). Finally, if collateral flow remains inadequate, arterial reconstruction with reversed interposition vein grafting is recommended. Most commonly, the cephalic, basilic, and saphenous veins are used as donor vessels. Resection of the damaged vessel is performed until patent side branches are encountered. Patency rates of more than 80% can be expected for this reconstruction.[10,11]

CONCLUSION

Vascular disorders of the upper extremity are relatively uncommon, but result in significant morbidity and functional loss. The physical examination findings and diagnostic tools to identify these disorders allow for their successful management.

REFERENCES

1. Coleman SS, Anson BJ. Arterial patterns in the hand based upon a study of 650 specimens. *Surg Gynecol Obstet.* 1961;113:409-424.

2. Kleinert JM, Fleming SG, Abel CS, Firrell J. Radial and ulnar artery dominance in normal digits. *J Hand Surg.* 1989;14A:504-508.

3. Phillips CS, Murphy MS. Vascular problems of the upper extremity: a primer for the orthopaedic surgeon. *J Am Acad Orthop Surg.* 2002;10(6):401-408.

4. Koman LA, Ruch DS, Smith BP, Smith TL. Vascular disorders of the hand. In: Green DP, Hotchkiss RN, Pederson WC, Wolfe SW (Ed). *Green's Operative Hand Surgery, Fifth Edition.* Philadelphia: Elsevier Churchill Livingstone; 2005:2265-2313.

5. Chloros GD, Smerlis NN, Li Z, et al. Noninvasive evaluation of upper-extremity vascular perfusion. *J Hand Surg.* 2008;33A:591-599.

6. Gelberman RH, Blasingame JP. The timed Allen test. *J Trauma.* 1981;21:477-479.

7. Ruch DS, Smith TL, Smith BP, et al. Anatomic and physiologic evaluation of upper extremity ischemia. *Microsurgery.* 1999;19:181-188.

8. Zimmerman NB. Occlusive vascular disorders of the upper extremity. *Hand Clin.* 1993;9:139-150.

9. Kleinert JM, Gupta A. Pulse volume recording. *Hand Clin.* 1993;9:13-46.

10. Zimmerman NB, Zimmerman SI, McClinton MA, et al. Long-term recovery following surgical treatment for ulnar artery occlusion. *J Hand Surg.* 1994;19A:17-21.

11. Koman LA, Urbaniak JR. Ulnar artery insufficiency: a guide to treatment. *J Hand Surg.* 1981;6:16-24.

12. Raskin KB. Acute vascular injuries of the upper extremity. *Hand Clin.* 1993;9:115-130.

FINANCIAL
DISCLOSURES

Dr. Brian D. Adams served as a consultant to Integra LifeSciences and Ascension Orthopedics.

Dr. Amy F. Austin has no financial or proprietary interest in the materials presented herein.

Dr. Taruna Madhav Crawford has no financial or proprietary interest in the materials presented herein.

Dr. Randall W. Culp has no financial or proprietary interest in the materials presented herein.

Dr. Seth D. Dodds receives an honorarium from Integra for educational lectures.

Dr. Jason M. Erpelding has no financial or proprietary interest in the materials presented herein.

Dr. David Essig has no financial or proprietary interest in the materials presented herein.

Dr. John Shum Sing Fai has no financial or proprietary interest in the materials presented herein.

Dr. John J. Fernandez has no financial or proprietary interest in the materials presented herein.

Dr. Jeffrey B. Friedrich has no financial or proprietary interest in the materials presented herein.

Dr. Sidney M. Jacoby has no financial or proprietary interest in the materials presented herein.

Dr. Hiu Yan Miranda Lai has not disclosed any relevant financial relationships.

Dr. Anthony J. Lauder is a consultant for Stryker.

Dr. Kristen E. McClure has no financial or proprietary interest in the materials presented herein.

Dr. William B. Morrison is a consultant and on the scientific board for GE Medical Systems and is a consultant for Apriomed Inc.

Dr. Frank E. Mullens has no financial or proprietary interest in the materials presented herein.

Dr. Min Jung Park has no financial or proprietary interest in the materials presented herein.

Dr. Diane Payne has no financial or proprietary interest in the materials presented herein.

Dr. Marc J. Richard has no financial or proprietary interest in the materials presented herein.

Dr. David Ring is a consultant for Wright Medical, Skeletal Dynamics, and Biomet and receives an honoraria from AO North America and AO International. He also receives royalties from Wright Medical and has contracted royalties with Biomet and Skeletal Dynamics and stock options with Illuminos. Dr. Ring receives funding for his Hand Surgery Fellowship from AO North America, and serves as Deputy Editor for *Review Articles, Journal of Hand Surgery, American*; Deputy Editor for *Hand and Wrist, Journal of Orthopaedic Trauma,* and Assistant Editor for the *Journal of Shoulder and Elbow Surgery.*

Dr. Danielle Scher has no financial or proprietary interest in the materials presented herein.

Dr. Uzoma Ukomadu has no financial or proprietary interest in the materials presented herein.

Dr. Brandon J. Valentine has no financial or proprietary interest in the materials presented herein.

Dr. Jennifer Moriatis Wolf is the Deputy Editor of *The Journal of Hand Surgery* and the Updates Editor for Vindico Medical Education and *Elsevier Skeletal Trauma.*

Dr. Jeffrey Yao is a consultant for Smith and Nephew Endoscopy and Arthrex and receives royalties from Arthrex.

INDEX

activity modification
  for arthritis, 267
  for cubital tunnel syndrome, 207
  for de Quervain's disease, 217
  for intersection syndrome, 219
  for medial epicondylitis, 225
  for pronator syndrome, 205–206
  for radial nerve compression, 209
  for ulnar tunnel syndrome, 206
adipofascial flap, 303
Adson's maneuver, 190, 197
Allen test, 32–33
  for Raynaud's phenomenon, 322–323
  for vascular disorders, 313–318
angiofibroblastic hyperplasia, 222
angiography, magnetic resonance
  of hand masses, 134
  of soft-tissue injuries and wounds, 298
  of vascular disorders, 324
anterior interosseous nerve syndrome, 192, 205–206
arteriography, contrast, 324–325
arteriovenous anastomosis, 322
arthritis, 252–253, 272. See also osteoarthritis; rheumatoid arthritis
  degenerative, 113–115
  of elbow, 88
  examination for, 254–264
  functional loss in, 253–254
  history of, 253–254
  imaging for, 129–131, 132, 265–267
  pathoanatomy of, 264–265

reactive/crystalline, 254
  treatment of, 267–271
arthrodesis
  for osteoarthritis of hand, 268
  radiolunate, 270
  for wrist ligament injuries, 173
arthrography, magnetic resonance
  of elbow, 76–77
  for ligament injury, 82, 103–105
  for osteochondral lesions, 87–88
  for ulnar wrist pain, 240
  of wrist, 98–99, 103–105
arthropathy, wrist, 111–115
arthroplasty
  of elbow, 271
  resectional, 268
  silicone implant, 268
  of ulnar head, 270
  for ulnar wrist pain, 246
  ulnohumeral, 271
  for wrist arthritis, 270
arthroscopy
  for arthritis of wrist, 267
  for ulnar wrist pain, 243, 245
auscultation, 313–318
autoimmune disease, evaluation for, 319–320
avascular necrosis, wrist, 117–118

bacterial colonization, 298
ballottement test
  for arthritis of hand, 259
  lunotriquetral, 28
  for ulnar wrist pain, 238
biceps brachii tendon injury, 83–84
biofeedback, for ulnar artery thrombosis, 326
blood flow, in hands, 311–312
bone scintigraphy
  for de Quervain's disease, 216

of elbow, 79, 92–93
  of hand, 125
  of wrist, 101
bone tumor
  of elbow, 91–93
  of hand, 134–135
Bouchard's nodes, 255
boutonnière deformity, 44, 257, 261
bowstringing deformity, 44
Boxer's fracture, 126
Buerger's disease, 324
Bunnell-Littler test, 57
burns, 293
bursitis, olecranon, 90

calcium-channel blockers, 326
capillary refill, 317
capitellum, osteochondral lesion of, 87
capitolunate instability, 173
capsular injuries of hand, 129
capsulodesis, dorsal, 172
carpal ligaments, 160
  injuries of, 161, 169–170
carpal shake test, 33, 34
carpal tunnel syndrome, 110–111, 186–187, 197–199
  imaging and tests for, 193–194, 203
  pathoanatomy of, 200
  treatment for, 203–205
carpometacarpal (CMC) joints, 49–51
  arthritis of, 255–260
cast immobilization, 173
cervical spine compression, 197
  tests for, 189–190
chair pick-up test, 221
claw hand deformity, 44, 62–63
closed fist test, 194
cold stress testing, 319
collateral ligament stress exam, 167

computed tomography (CT)
  for coronoid fractures, 283
  for distal humerus fracture, 284
  of elbow, 74–76
    for arthritis, 88
    for instability, 153–154
    for soft-tissues masses, 93
    for trauma, 80
    for tumor, 91
  for forearm fractures, 285
  of hand, 122
    for foreign body, 135–136
    for fracture, 125
  for scaphoid fractures, 282
  of soft-tissue injuries and wounds, 298
  for ulnar wrist pain, 239–240
  for vascular disorders, 324
  of wrist, 96, 103
coronoid fractures
  examination for, 278, 283–284
  O'Driscoll classification of, 153
  treatment of, 155
crepitation, 275
cross-finger flap, 303–304
cross-finger test, 62
crush injury, 295
cubital tunnel compression, 184
cubital tunnel syndrome
  imaging, 85–86
  tests for, 194–195, 199
  treatment for, 207–209

Darrach procedure, 270
de Quervain's disease
  in arthritis of hand, 260
  examination for, 215
  history of, 213–215
  imaging for, 216
  pathoanatomy of, 216
  treatment of, 217–218
deformity
  in fracture assessment, 275
  in hand fractures, 287–288
diabetes mellitus, 312
digital brachial index, 319

disease-modifying anti-rheumatic drugs (DMARDs), 267–268
dislocations, in ischemia of fingers, 321
distal interphalangeal (DIP) joint
  arthritis of, 253, 255, 261, 268
  stiffness of, 177
distal radioulnar joint (DRUJ)
  arthritis of, 25
  injuries of, 228–229
    diagnosis of, 232–240
    examination for, 169
    helpful hints for managing, 178
    pathoanatomy of, 229–232
    treatment of, 241–248
  instability of
    examination for, 278, 281
    imaging of, 171–172
    tests for, 25
  pathoanatomy of, 170
Doppler vascular examination, 316, 318–319
double crush phenomenon, 186, 201
Durkan's compression maneuver, 193, 197–199

Eichoff maneuver, 215
elbow
  arthritis of
    imaging for, 88–89, 267
    treatment for, 271
  atrophy of mobile wad of three, 4–5
  bone and cartilage pathology of, 87–88
  bony deformity of, 4
  compression neuropathies of, 185
  detailed history of, 2–3
  dislocations of, 149
    examination for, 276–279
    proximal radioulnar joint, 151
    radial head, 150–151
    treatment of, 155
  effusion at, 75
  fracture-dislocations of, 152
    treatment of, 155
    imaging of, 73–93

infection of, 88–90
instability of, 139, 155–156
  classification of, 140–142
  examination for, 143–150
  history of, 143
  imaging of, 153–154
  pathoanatomy of, 150–153
  treatment of, 154–155
  intra-articular bodies in, 75
  masses in, 91–93
  muscle injuries of, 83–84
  normal carrying angle of, 5
  overuse injuries of, 80–82
  physical examination of, 3, 13
    palpation, 6–9
    provocative maneuver/special tests, 9–12
    range of motion, 6
    strength testing, 8–9
    visual inspection, 3–5
  posterolateral rotary instability of, 12
  psoriatic lesions of, 3
  regions of, 150
  soft spots along, 4
  swelling, 3
  tendopathies of, 212, 220–226
  terrible triad, 152–153
  trauma to
    imaging for, 79–80
    signs of, 3
  ulnar neuropathy of, 85–87
elbow flexion tests, 195, 285
electromyography (EMG), 201–203
elevated fat pad sign, 79–80
epicondylectomy, 225
epicondylitis
  elbow tenderness in, 7
  lateral, 80–81, 214, 220–223
  medial, 9, 80–81, 214, 223–225
Esssex-Lopresti lesions, 229
excision, for osteoarthritis of hand, 268
extensor carpi ulnaris (ECU) subluxation test, 28, 29, 235

extensor digitorum communis tendons, 23–24

fasciocutaneous flaps, 307–308
finger nail clubbing, 42
finger/thumb extension loss, 195
fingers
    active-passive mismatch in, 55–56
    blood flow in, 312
    fractures of, 287–289
    goniometric measurement of, 54–56
    ischemia of, 321–324
    loss of flexion of, 56–57
    open wounds of, 303–304
Finkelstein test, 19, 215
fixation
    for elbow instability, 154, 155
    for hand ligament injuries, 176–177
    open reduction and internal
        for hand ligament injuries, 176–177
        for ulnar wrist pain, 241
        for scapholunate rupture, 172–173
flap closures, of soft-tissue injuries, 303–308
flexor carpi radialis tendon
    tenderness of, 29
    tendinopathy of, 219–220
flexor pulley injury, 128
flexor superficialis testing, 57, 58
fluorodeoxyglucose positron emission tomography, 93
forearm
    compression neuropathies of, 185
    fractures of, 285–287
    mangling injury of, 307–308
    open wounds of, 308
foreign body, in hand, 135–136
fractures
    of elbow, 152–153
    examination for, 274–289
    of fingers, 127
    of hand, 125–126, 287–289
    inspection for, 274–275
    in ischemia of fingers, 321
    lunate, 20

patient history of, 275–276
radial head, 279–281
scaphoid, 278, 281, 282
through enchondroma, 134
of wrist, 101–102, 281, 282–285
free-flap reconstruction, 295
free muscle flaps, 307–308
free-tissue transfer, 307–308
Froment's sign, 61, 194

Galeazzi fractures, 229–230
gamekeeper's thumb, 129
giant cell tumor
    of elbow, 91
    of tendon sheath, 133–134
glumus, 322
grafts, for elbow instability, 154
granulation tissue, 296, 298, 299
grind test
    for arthritis of hand, 256, 260
    of carpometacarpal joints, 18, 50
    pisotriquetral, 257
grip-and-pinch strength testing, 59–60
grip function, 38, 39
grip testing, 9, 33–34
Guyon's canal. See ulnar tunnel syndrome

hamate fracture, 31–32
hand
    arthritis of
        examination for, 255–261
        imaging, 265
        treatment for, 268
    capillary refill assessment in, 46
    causes of deformity in, 43
    deformities of, 42–44
    edema of, 44–45
    fractures of, 287–289
    functional loss in, 38
    imaging of, 121
        clinical indications for, 125–136
        modalities of, 122–125
    innervation of, 67–70
    joint pain in, 47–48
    joint stability of, 48
    ligament injuries of, 159, 177–179
        examination for, 167–168, 174–175

imaging of, 175–176
    pathoanatomy of, 175
    patient history, 173–174
    treatment of, 176–177
ligament stability in, 52
mangling injury of, 305
microvascular beds of, 311
muscle atrophy in, 45–46
open wounds of, 304–307
patient history, 37–38
physical examination of
    inspection in, 40–45
    palpation in, 45–51
    preliminary, 36–40
    range of motion in, 52–59, 60
    sensory testing in, 66–70
    strength testing in, 59–66, 60
    surface anatomy, 51–52
sensory patterns in, 198
skin assessment of, 41, 42, 46
skin creases in, 53
vascular anatomy of, 311–312
hand-based flaps, 304
Heberden's nodes, 255, 256
hemangioma, 322
heterodigital flaps, 303–304
homodigital flaps, 303
hourglass at dorsal wrist, 258
humerus fractures, distal, 284
hypothenar hammer syndrome, 322

imaging
    for arthritis
        of elbow, 267
        of hand, 265
        of wrist, 265–266
    for compression neuropathy, 201–203
    for de Quervain's disease, 216
    of elbow, 73, 79–93, 153–154
        modalities of, 74–78
    for epicondylitis, lateral and medial, 222, 225
    pitfalls of, 101
    for soft-tissue injuries and wounds, 298
    for ulnar wrist pain, 238–240

for vascular disorders, 324–325
of wrist, 95–118
for ligament injuries, 170–172
modalities of, 96–101
immobilization
for hand ligament injuries, 177
for ulnar wrist pain, 243–245
implant arthroplasty, ulnar, 247–248
infection
of elbow, 88–91
forearm wound following, 306
of hand, 132–133
of soft tissue, 292–293
injection test, in compression neuropathy, 195
interosseous artery flap, posterior, 306
interosseous nerves
anterior, palsy of, 186
posterior
neuroma of, 24
pathology of, 195–196, 199, 209
interosseous syndrome, 186–187
interphalangeal joints, 49
intersection syndrome, 19–20, 214, 218–219

joint active-passive mismatch, 55–56
joint effusion/recesses, wrist, 115–116

Kasabach-Merritt syndrome, 322
keloid scars, 300
Kienböck disease, 20
Kienböck's necrosis, wrist, 117–118

Lachman test, 149
lateral collateral ligament repair, 154
Leiche sympathectomy, 326
Lichtman midcarpal shift test, 161, 165
grading system for, 169
lift-off test, 146, 149
ligament injuries
of hand, 129, 159, 177–179
examination for, 167–168, 174–175
imaging of, 175–176

pathoanatomy of, 175
patient history, 173–174
treatment of, 176–177
with radial head fractures, 279
of wrist, 159–160, 177–179
examination for, 161–169
imaging for, 103–108, 170–172
pathoanatomy of, 169–170
patient history, 160–161
treatment of, 172–173
Linscheid's test, 23, 51, 52
lunate fracture, 20
lunotriquetral disruption, 160
lunotriquetral ligament injuries, 27–28, 171

Madelung's deformity, 229
magnetic resonance imaging (MRI)
for biceps brachii tendon injury, 83–84
for compression neuropathy, 201–202
for cubital tunnel syndrome, 85–86
for de Quervain's disease, 216
of elbow, 78–80, 88
for osteomyelitis, 90
for soft-tissues masses, 93
for tumors, 91–92
of hand, 123–125
for arthritis, 129–131
for bone tumor, 135
for foreign bodies, 136
for fractures, 125
for infection, 132–133
for ligament and capsular injuries, 129
for soft tissue masses, 133–134
for tendon injury, 126–127
for medial and lateral epicondylitis, 81, 222, 225
for osteochondral lesions, 87–88
for pulley injuries, 127–128
for soft-tissue injuries and wounds, 298
for triceps tendon injury, 84

for ulnar collateral ligament injury, 82
for ulnar nerve dislocation and snapping triceps syndrome, 86–87
of wrist, 100
for arthritis, 267
for arthropathy, 111–113
for avascular necrosis, 117–118
for joint effusion/recesses, 115–116
for ligament injuries, 105–108, 171
for tendinopathy, 108–110
for trauma, 103
for tumors and masses, 116–117
for ulnar pain, 240
malignancy, upper extremity, 293
mallet deformity, 44
masses
of elbow, 91–93
soft-tissue, 296
of wrist, 116–117
median nerve
compression of, 30, 186–187
motor tests for, 198
treatment for, 203–206
sensory patterns for, 198
metacarpophalangeal (MCP) joint, 48–49
arthritis of, 255
injuries to, 173–174
imaging of, 176
pathoanatomy of, 175
treatment of, 176–177
midcarpal instability, 27, 160
palmar, 173
middle finger test, 195
milking maneuver, 9, 11
motor testing, nerve-specific, 198
mucous cyst, hand, 256
muscle
injuries of in elbow, 83–84
strength grading system for, 60–61

nerve conduction studies, 201–203
neuromas, wrist, 111
neuropathy
compression, 183–184, 209–210
causes of, 184

imaging/testing for, 201–203
morbidity and prevalence of, 184
motor tests for, 198
pathoanatomy of, 199–201
patient history, 184–188
physical examination for, 188–199
risk factors for, 186
sensory changes in, 197
symptoms of, 186
treatment of, 203–209
of wrist, 110–111
neurovascular examination, 275
nuclear medicine scans. See bone scintigraphy

occlusive disease
in ischemia of fingers, 322
post-traumatic, 326
OK procedure, 271
"okay" sign, 63–64
olecranon, osteomyelitis of, 88–90
opera glass hand, 261
osteoarthritis, 252–253, 254
of elbow, 267
imaging of, 267
erosive, 255
of hand, 256, 258–259
pathoanatomy of, 264
pisotriquetral, 257
of wrist, 261–263
treatment of, 269–270
osteoarthropathy, elbow, 88
osteochondral lesions, 87–88
osteomyelitis, 88–90
overuse injuries, 212–213. See also tendinopathy
of elbow, 80–82
in ulnar wrist pain, 233

palpation
of fractures, 275
for vascular disorders, 313–318
paratendonitis, 213
Parsonage-Turner syndrome, 205
pedicled groin flap, 306–307
perilunate dislocations, 172
perilunate instability, 169
peripheral nerve, organization of, 200

peripheral nervous system, vascular control by, 312
Phalen's test, 30, 193, 197–199
physical examination
for elbow dislocation, 276–279
for elbow instability, 143–150
for forearm fractures, 285–287
for fractures, 274–289
of hand, 287–289
of radial head, 279–281
of wrist, 281, 282–285
for soft-tissue injuries and wounds, 293–296
for vascular disorders, 313–320
physical therapy
for lateral epicondylitis, 222
for tendonitis, 214
piano key test, 25
for arthritis of hand, 260
for DRUJ injuries, 166
for ulnar wrist pain, 234, 242
pinch meter, 65–66
pinch strength testing, 9, 65–66
pisiform boost test, 237
pisiform shear test, 31
pisotriquetral arthritis, 31
pivot-shift apprehension test, 144, 149
plethysmography, digital, 319
point tenderness, 195
positron emission tomography, 93
posterior interosseous nerve syndrome
testing for, 195–196, 199
treatment of, 209
posterolateral rotatory drawer test, 145, 149
power grip, 38
precision grip, 38, 39
pressure dressings, 302
pronation test, 196
pronator syndrome, 8, 9, 186–187
testing for, 192
treatment for, 205–206
proximal interphalangeal (PIP) joint
arthritis of, 255
dislocation of, 178

injuries to, 173–174
examination of, 174
imaging of, 175–176
pathoanatomy of, 175
treatment of, 176–177
proximal interphalangeal (PIP) joint stress exam, 167
pulley injuries, 127–128
pulse volume recordings, 319
push-off test, 34

radial collateral ligament injury, 174
examination for, 174–175
imaging of, 176
treatment of, 177
radial forearm flap, 304–306
radial head fractures, 279–281
radial nerve
compression of, 188
motor tests for, 198
treatment for, 209
sensory patterns for, 198
testing muscles of, 64–65
radial tunnel syndrome, 9, 188
tests for, 195–196, 199
treatment for, 209
radiography
for arthritis, 265–267
for biceps brachii tendon injury, 83
for bone tumor of hand, 134–135
for compression neuropathy, 201
for cubital tunnel syndrome, 86
for de Quervain's disease, 216
for distal humerus fracture, 284
of elbow, 74
for arthritis, 88
for instability, 148, 153–154
for osteomyelitis, 90
for soft-tissues masses, 93
for trauma, 79–80
for tumors, 91
for flexor carpi radialis tendinopathy, 220
of hand, 122
for arthritis, 129–131

for foreign body, 135–136
for fracture, 125–126
for infection, 132–133
for soft tissue masses, 133–134
for intersection syndrome, 219
for medial and lateral epicondylitis, 81, 222, 225
for osteochondral lesions, 87–88
for reflex sympathetic dystrophy, 131
for triceps tendon injury, 84
for ulnar collateral ligament injury, 82
for ulnar nerve dislocation and snapping triceps syndrome, 86
of wrist, 96, 97–98
for arthropathy, 111–112, 114
for avascular necrosis, 117–118
for ligament injuries, 103–105, 170–171
for trauma, 101–103
for ulnar pain, 238–239
radioulnar ligament injuries, 161
radius fractures, distal, 282–283
radius-pull test, 283
range of motion
of elbow, 6
of hand, 52–59, 60
of wrist, 15
rapport, establishing with patient, 3
Raynaud's disease, 321, 323
Raynaud's phenomenon, 322–323
reflex sympathetic dystrophy, of hand, 131
relocation test, 237
repetitive insults, vascular, 313
resistance testing, 192
rheumatoid arthritis, 252–253, 254
of elbow, 88, 89
treatment of, 271
of hand, 261
examination for, 256–257, 258–260
imaging of, 130

pathoanatomy of, 264–265
treatment of, 267–268
of wrist, 263–264
imaging, 111–112
treatment of, 269–270
rheumatoid nodules, 257, 261
ring finger malunion, 288

Sauvé-Kapandji procedure, 246–247, 269
scaphoid fractures, 278, 281, 282
scaphoid nonunion advanced collapse (SNAC) wrists, 266–267
scaphoid ring sign, 171
scaphoid thrust (Lane) test, 23
scapholunate
dissociation of, 16–17, 21, 160, 178
instability of, 22
pain in, 161
rupture of, 172–173
scapholunate advanced collapse (SLAC) wrist, 261–262
imaging for, 265–266
scapholunate interval, 20–21
scaphotrapezial joint arthritis, 18
scar contracture, 296
examination for, 294
treatment of, 298–301
scarring
after crush injury, 295
examination for, 294
with free-flap reconstruction, 295
with wound healing, 296–297
segmental arterial pressures, 316, 319
Semmes-Weinstein monofilament, 69–70, 197
Semmes-Weinstein monofilament test, 191
sensory radial nerve compression, 209
sensory testing, hand, 66–70
septic arthritis
of hand, 132
of wrist, 112–113
shear test, 259
shift test
midcarpal, 161, 164
grading system for, 169

scaphoid (Watson's), 22–23, 258
shuck test, 28
lunotriquetral, 163
thumb carpometacarpal joint, 50–51
sitting hands test, 33, 34
skin grafts, 301, 303–308
skin malignancy, excision of, 302
snapping triceps syndrome, 86–87
soft-tissue envelope, 291–292
assessment of, 293–296
soft tissue injuries, 291–292
closure of, 301–302
examination for, 293–296
imaging for, 298
pathoanatomy of, 296–298
patient history of, 292–293
treatment of, 298–308
soft tissue masses
of elbow, 93
of hand, 133–134
soft-tissue rebalancing, 268
splinting
for arthritis, 267
for cubital tunnel syndrome, 207
for de Quervain's disease, 217
for flexor carpi radialis tendinopathy, 220
for intersection syndrome, 219
for lateral epicondylitis, 222
for median nerve compression, 203
for radial nerve compression, 209
for wrist ligament injuries, 173
Spurling's maneuver, 189, 197
squeeze test, 28
stability testing, elbow, 9–11
Stener lesion, 129
stenosing flexor tenosynovitis, 255
steroids
for arthritis, 267
for de Quervain's disease, 217
for flexor carpi radialis tendinopathy, 220

for lateral epicondylitis, 223

for median nerve compression, 203–204

strength testing
of elbow, 8–9
of hand, 59–66, 60

stress testing
of hand ligaments, 51
MCP joint, 167–168

subclavian artery, 311

Sudeck's atrophy, 131

surgical decompression
for flexor carpi radialis tendinopathy, 220
for intersection syndrome, 219
for median nerve compression, 203–205

surgical interventions
for arthritis of elbow, 271
for cubital tunnel syndrome, 207–209
for de Quervain's disease, 217–218
for elbow instability, 154–155
for lateral epicondylitis, 223, 224
for medial epicondylitis, 225
for osteoarthritis of hand, 268
for osteoarthritis of wrist, 269–270
for radial nerve compression, 209, 210
for ulnar wrist pain, 241, 243–245

surgical resection, vascular, 326

swan neck deformity, 44, 257, 261

synovectomy, 271

synovitis, 33

table press test, 169

tabletop relocation test, 147, 149

tendinopathy, 212–226
with trigger finger, 128
of wrist, 108–110

tendinosis, 213

tendon injury, hand, 126–127

tendon transfers, 268

tendonitis, 212–213
of extensor digitorum communis tendons, 23–24

FCR, 214
of FCU tendon, 32
in radial dorsal wrist pain, 19
tests for, 9
of ulnar dorsal wrist, 28

tennis elbow, 220–223

tenosynovectomy, 268

tenosynovitis
de Quervain's, 19
of hand, 133
in radial dorsal wrist pain, 19
in rheumatoid arthritis, 263–264
of second dorsal extensor, 19–20
of ulnar dorsal wrist, 28

Terry Thomas sign, 171

thenar flap, 304

thermal injury, 293

thoracic outlet compression test, 189–190, 197

thoracic outlet syndrome, 197

threshold testing, 69–70

thromboangiitis obliterans, 324

thumb
CMC instability test of, 19
dorsal avulsion injury of, 305
MCP stress exam of, 167
metacarpophalangeal joint radial collateral ligament injury of, 178
metacarpophalangeal joint ulnar collateral ligament injury of, 178
retropulsion of, 64–65

thumb spica short arm cast, 177

Tinel's sign, 7–8
in compression neuropathy, 188
in elbow fractures, 285

Tinel's test
for compression neuropathy, 188, 190
for cubital tunnel syndrome, 199
in Guyon's canal, 32
for nerve compression, 197
over dorsal sensory radial nerve, 20
for wrist nerve compression, 30

touch sensation, 69

traction, 176

trampoline test, 236

trauma
in compression neuropathy, 199–200
to elbow, 79–80, 143
to hand, 125–129
in ischemia of fingers, 321
to soft-tissue envelope, 292
in ulnar wrist pain, 229
in vascular disorders, 326
in vascular injury, 312
to wrist, 101–103

triangular fibrocartilage, arthritis of, 267

triangular fibrocartilage complex (TFCC)
injuries to, 25–26, 169, 228–229
diagnosis of, 232–240
Palmer classification of, 231–232
pathoanatomy of, 229–232
treatment of, 241–248
tears of
helpful hints for managing, 178
imaging, 103–108
traumatic tears to, 160–161

triangular fibrocartilage complex (TFCC) load test, 26

triceps tendon injury, 84

trigger finger, 127, 128, 255

tumors
soft-tissue, 296
of upper extremity, 293
of wrist, 116–117

two-point discrimination test
for compression neuropathy, 191
for fractures, 275

ulna
displaced fracture of, 286–287
impaction lesion of, 236

ulnar artery, 311
thrombosis of, 326

ulnar collateral ligament injury, 82, 174
imaging of, 176
pathoanatomy of, 175
treatment of, 177

ulnar compression test, 237, 242

ulnar drift, 256
ulnar fovea sign (Berger's), 32–33, 161
ulnar fovea test, 164
ulnar head resection, 246
ulnar nerve, 67
  compression neuropathies of, 185
  compression of, 184, 187–188
  motor tests for, 198
  treatment for, 206–209
  dislocation of, 86–87
  dysfunction of with elbow fractures, 285
  injuries to, strength testing for, 63
  pathologies of, 7–8
  sensory patterns for, 198
ulnar neuropathy
  imaging, 85–87
  tests for, 9
ulnar recession, 245–246
ulnar shortening procedure
  for ulnar wrist pain, 245–246
  for wrist ligament injuries, 173
ulnar tunnel syndrome, 206–207
ulnocarpal stress test, 166, 234
ulnotriquetral ligament injuries, 161
ultrasound
  for biceps brachii tendon injury, 83
  for cubital tunnel syndrome, 86
  for de Quervain's disease, 216
  of elbow, 77–78
  for arthritis, 88
  for osteomyelitis, 90
  for soft-tissues masses, 93
  of hand, 122–123
  for arthritis, 131
  for foreign body, 135
  for fracture, 125
  for infection, 132
  for ligament and capsular injuries, 129
  for soft tissue masses, 133–134

for tendon injury, 126–127
for medial and lateral epicondylitis, 81, 222
for pulley injuries, 127–128
for triceps tendon injury, 84
for ulnar collateral ligament injury, 82
for ulnar nerve dislocation and snapping triceps syndrome, 86–87
for vascular disorders, 316, 318–319
of wrist, 99
  for arthropathy, 111, 113, 115
  for avascular necrosis, 117–118
  for joint effusion/recesses, 115–116
  for neuropathy, 110–111
  for tendinopathy, 108–110

valgus extension overload test, 10
valgus instability, post-traumatic, 151
varus stress test, 283
vascular anatomy, 311–312
vascular disorders, 310
  evaluation for, 313–320
  imaging in, 324–325
  pathoanatomy in, 320–324
  patient history of, 312–313
  treatment of, 325–326
venous thoracic outlet syndrome, 3
vibratory testing, 69–70
vitamin B6, 203
volar intercalated segmental instability (VISI), 170, 173

wafer procedure, 245–246
Wartenberg's syndrome, 20, 196, 209
Watson's/scaphoid shift test, 162
wounds
  drainage pf, 299
  healing of, 296–297
  open

examination of, 294, 295–296
management of, 299–300
pathoanatomy of, 296–298
treatment of, 301–308
Wright's maneuver, 189, 197
wrist
  arthritis of
    examination for, 261–264
    imaging, 265–267
    treatment for, 269–270
  central dorsal zone of, 20–24
  compression neuropathies of, 185
  fractures of, 281, 282–285
  imaging of, 95, 101–118
    modalities of, 96–101
  instability of, 22, 260
  ligament injuries of, 159–160, 177–179
    examination for, 161–169
    imaging for, 170–172
    pathoanatomy of, 169–170
    patient history, 160–161
    treatment of, 172–173
  physical examination of, 14–15, 35
    general tests, 32–34
    history, 15
    inspection/palpation, 15–16
    topographic, 16–32
  radial dorsal zone of, 16–20
  radial volar zone of, 28–30
  repetitive hyperextension of, 18
  snuffbox, 17–18
  tendinopathies of, 212–220, 225–226
  ulnar dorsal zone of, 24–28
  ulnar pain in, 228–248
  ulnar volar zone of, 30–32

x-ray, wrist, 235

Z-plasty, 300–301

Printed in the United States
by Baker & Taylor Publisher Services

Printed in the United States
by Baker & Taylor Publisher Services